ADULT PALLIATIVE CARE
FOR NURSING, HEALTH
AND SOCIAL CARE

EDITED BY
JOHN COSTELLO

ADULT PALLIATIVE CARE FOR NURSING, HEALTH AND SOCIAL CARE

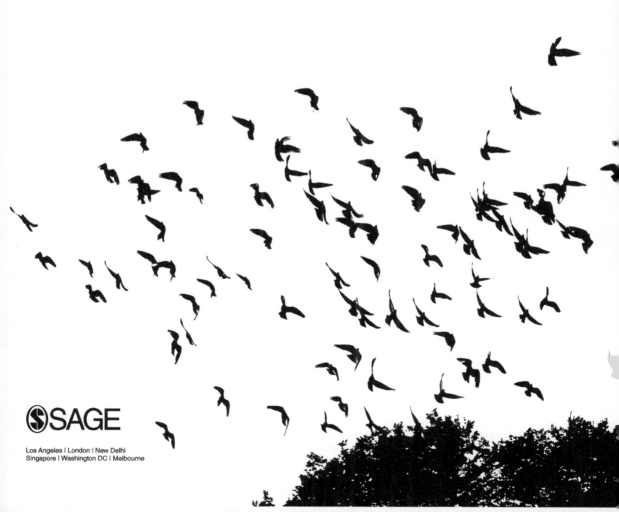

⑩SAGE

Los Angeles | London | New Delhi
Singapore | Washington DC | Melbourne

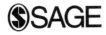

Los Angeles | London | New Delhi
Singapore | Washington DC | Melbourne

SAGE Publications Ltd
1 Oliver's Yard
55 City Road
London EC1Y 1SP

SAGE Publications Inc.
2455 Teller Road
Thousand Oaks, California 91320

SAGE Publications India Pvt Ltd
B 1/I 1 Mohan Cooperative Industrial Area
Mathura Road
New Delhi 110 044

SAGE Publications Asia-Pacific Pte Ltd
3 Church Street
#10-04 Samsung Hub
Singapore 049483

Editor: Alex Clabburn
Editorial assistant: Jade Grogan
Production editor: Victoria Nicholas
Marketing manager: Tamara Navaratnam
Cover design: Wendy Scott
Typeset by: C&M Digitals (P) Ltd, Chennai, India
Printed in the UK

Library of Congress Control Number: 2018941830

British Library Cataloguing in Publication data

A catalogue record for this book is available from
the British Library

ISBN 978-1-5264-0836-5
ISBN 978-1-5264-0837-2 (pbk)

At SAGE we take sustainability seriously. Most of our products are printed in the UK using responsibly sourced
papers and boards. When we print overseas we ensure sustainable papers are used as measured by the
PREPS grading system. We undertake an annual audit to monitor our sustainability.

CONTENTS

ABOUT THE EDITOR AND CONTRIBUTORS

EDITOR

Dr John Costello is an honorary lecturer at the University of Manchester, School of Nursing, Midwifery and Social Work. Before this, he was a senior lecturer in palliative care at the school. John has been a teacher of palliative care at undergraduate and postgraduate levels for over 30 years. His research interests focus on the social management of death, dying and bereavement. He has published extensively on these topics nationally and internationally, authoring four books and over a hundred research articles. He remains research active and continues to make a contribution to academic research.

CONTRIBUTORS

Joan Smith is a retired health service manager, lecturer and patient on dialysis.

Josephine Pople is a staff nurse at Wythenshawe Hospital, Manchester University NHS Foundation Trust.

Sharon Grimsdale is a community heart failure nurse specialist at Bradford Teaching Hospitals NHS Foundation Trust.

Susan Heatley is matron/lead for palliative and end of life care at Central Manchester University Hospitals NHS Foundation Trust.

Jacqueline Crowther is an Honorary Research Associate at the University of Liverpool and is an Admiral Nurse at Kirkwood Hospice.

Ahamed Ashique is medical director of the Hospital Palliative Care Team at Central Manchester Hospital Foundation Trust.

Anne Golden is a specialist palliative care social worker.

Andrew Bradley is the chaplaincy and spiritual care coordinator at the Christie Hospital NHS Foundation Trust.

Anne-Marie Raftery is clinical lead and Macmillan clinical nurse specialist in palliative care at The Christie NHS Foundation Trust.

Carole Farrell is a teaching fellow/honorary lecturer in the Division of Nursing, Midwifery and Social Work, School of Health Sciences, Faculty of Biology, Medicine and Health at The University of Manchester.

Alison Newey is a COPD Specialist Nursing Service Lead.

ACKNOWLEDGEMENTS

The author and publisher would like to thank everyone who provided case material from their personal and professional experience for the chapters, including Jeff and Sue Edwards; the book is much richer for your contributions.

Thanks also to artist Betty Dewey for providing drawings for the chapters.

We would also like to thank the lecturers and practice professionals who helped to shape and impact the book's development at crucial stages:

Peter Ellis

Peter Jones

Deborah Maclaren

Michael McGivern

Janice Pearson

INTRODUCTION

In the last decade, the amount of literature, research and government policy highlighting the needs of patients at the end of life and their families, to receive expert care and treatment has grown significantly. In July 2016, the UK Government made a new National Commitment on end of life care (Department of Health, 2016) which was the most comprehensive and significant policy announcement for palliative and end of life care since the 2008 strategy, affecting health care interventions made in hospitals and community settings in relation to palliative and end of life care:

> Our commitment is that every person nearing the end of their life should receive attentive, high quality, compassionate care, so that their pain is eased, their spirits lifted and their wishes for their closing weeks, days and hours are respected – Ben Gummer MP, Parliamentary Under Secretary for Care Quality 2015–16.

Moreover, the NICE guidance (2017) on end of life care, if implemented, should contribute significantly towards improving end of life care and lead to a greater focus on non-cancer conditions. These initiatives have helped in the writing of this book, which takes a non-standard approach to palliative care provision by shifting attention onto the care of people with non-cancer conditions.

The aim of this book is to raise the awareness of healthcare professionals working in palliative care of the experiences of those families and patients on the palliative care journey. It does this by giving a voice to patients and families and encouraging them to amplify their experiences in the chapters of this book. The book is divided into two parts: **Part 1 Palliative Care Practice** focuses on a description of different life-limiting conditions and the care and treatment patients require during the palliative and end of life phases of their illnesses. **Part 2 Support for Families and Caregivers** focuses on the supportive aspects of palliative care for families and caregivers.

Chapter 1 The experience of living with cancer by Joan Smith, a patient living with cancer, focuses on her experiences of living with her diagnosis, along with the effects of treatment which she recalls in an extended case study.

Chapter 2 Palliative care for people with end stage pulmonary disease by Josephine Pople, who has a background in respiratory nursing with a focus on palliative care, provides a comprehensive account of the transition from acute respiratory failure to the situation where patients and families require specialist palliative care, as the patient's condition deteriorates.

Chapter 3 Palliative care for people with end stage heart failure (ESHF) by Sharon Grimsdale, a clinical nurse specialist in heart failure, considers patients with End Stage Heart Failure and their journey from early diagnosis to end of life and the treatments and nursing care provided to the patient, as well as the support provided to family caregivers.

Together with colleagues from the MS Society UK and patients with MS, I wrote **Chapter 4 Palliative care for people with multiple sclerosis which considers** the complex case of patients with Multiple Sclerosis who spend most of their lives outside of hospital but reach a stage where they require palliative and end of life care.

Chapter 5 Patients with end stage renal failure by Susan Heatley, a Matron and lead nurse in palliative care, describes the palliative care journey of patients with renal disease. Susan develops a dual perspective on End Stage Renal Disease, looking at the nursing perspective alongside a contribution by Joan Smith from **Chapter 1.**

Chapter 6 Palliative care for people with advanced dementia by Jacqueline Crowther, a specialist Admiral Nurse in Dementia care, focuses attention on the care of people with dementia using personal and academic views of the care of the patient and the support provided to family caregivers.

Part II Support for Families and Caregivers begins with **Chapter 7 Symptom management: the medical perspective** by Ahamed Ashique, a medical consultant in palliative care, and myself provides an overview of the medical perspective and symptom management of patients who require palliative care treatment. We give an account of the medical management of patients from diagnosis to death, focusing on the importance of team-working, accurate patient assessment and sensitive psychological support for families and lay caregivers.

Chapter 8 Supporting families and lay caregivers on the palliative care journey by Anne Golden, a specialist palliative care social worker, considers the supportive care aspects of helping patients and families who experience many complex and varied situations in their palliative care journey, as well as bereavement after care issues.

Chapter 9 Grief, bereavement and spirituality, is a joint endeavour between Andrew Bradley and myself. Andrew contributes his experiences as a spiritual care coordinator in a large oncology hospital. Together we take a sensitive view of the end of life experiences of patients and families, as well as discussing bereavement after care.

Chapter 10 Ethical dilemmas in palliative care is written by Anne-Marie Raftery, a Macmillan Cancer Nurse, and Carole Farrell, Nurse and AHP Research Fellow, who examine the ethical issues that invariably occur when patients are receiving palliative care. They help us to consider some of the complexities associated with breaking bad news and some of the sensitive aspects of end of life care.

Chapter 11 Hospital palliative care teams by Anne-Marie Raftery gives an account of the role of hospital palliative care teams in supporting practitioners within a hospital context.

Finally, **Chapter 12 End of life care in the community** by Alison Newey, a COPD Specialist Nursing Service Lead, gives a comprehensive account of end of life care in a community context.

Most of the chapters utilise real-life case studies with consent from patients and families to share their experiences with a wider professional audience. Their experiences should help readers develop greater insights into palliative care practice. Moreover, students will find the book useful for increasing their evidence-based knowledge of palliative care and educators will find it a valuable resource for teaching the holistic care of patients with a wide range of life-limiting illnesses, not just cancer. It is a book aimed at not just improving knowledge of palliative care but informing and improving practice by contributing to our awareness of the palliative care journey from diagnosis to death. By hearing patients and caregiver's stories, students and professionals should be able to improve quality of life by developing effective practice based on sound, informed clinical insights.

REFERENCES

Department of Health (2016) *Our Commitment to you for end of life care.* London: Department of Health.

NICE Pathways (2017) *End of life care for people with life-limiting conditions.* London: NICE. Available at: https://pathways.nice.org.uk/pathways/end-of-life-care-for-people-with-life-limiting-conditions, accessed March 2017.

PART I

PALLIATIVE CARE PRACTICE

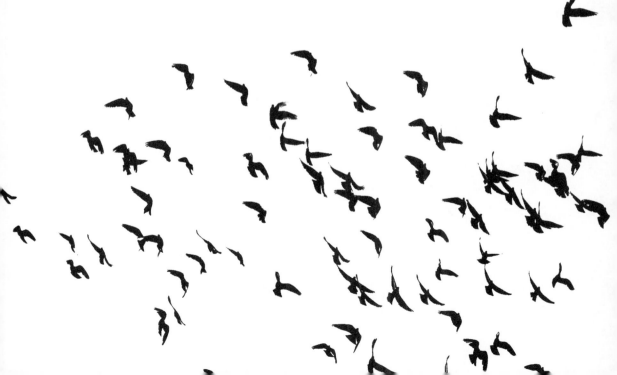

1

THE EXPERIENCE OF LIVING WITH CANCER

JOAN SMITH

LEARNING OUTCOMES

- Become aware of how a cancer diagnosis impacts on service users/patients and those who are important to them
- Be able to consider the implications of the cancer experience
- Have the opportunity to reflect on their professional relationship with patients who have cancer
- Recognise the importance of empathy in the management of patients with a life-limiting illness

INTRODUCTION

There are an increasing number of people surviving cancer (Macmillan, 2013), although evidence suggests that these survivors do not always have their personal needs met by professionals. Moreover, it has been reported that one in three cancer survivors find that many of their needs for cancer treatment and care go unmet (Morgan, 2009). These findings are supported by National Patient Reported Outcomes Measures (PROMs) which found that post cancer treatment patients had poorer quality of life scores when compared to the general population (Glaser et al., 2013). This chapter therefore focuses on the important perspective of the patient, focusing on the author's personal experience of cancer.

It begins with background information on the incidence, causation and epidemiology of cancer diagnosis in the UK, highlighting the most common cancers. It also looks briefly at some of the causes of cancer while recognising that not all cancers have known causes. The chapter looks at how nurses and others can help and support the patient throughout the treatment as well as post treatment and how the individual can help take control of their life after cancer treatment. Because the chapter reflects on personal experience, use of the first person pronoun 'I' will be used throughout as it reflects on the writer's personal experience from the initial diagnosis, through treatment and then describes coming to terms with the impact cancer had on her life.

INCIDENCE OF CANCER

Cancer Research UK (2016a) estimates that, for those born after 1960, one in two will develop cancer at some stage of their life. A common misconception about cancer is that a cancer diagnosis means a terminal illness. However, as the evidence suggests, more and more people are surviving cancer. The cancer charity Macmillan (2013) has stated that in 2013 there were 2.5 million people living with cancer in the UK and this was projected to rise to 4 million by 2030. At the same time, Macmillan's Recovery Package (2013) identifies positive steps that can be taken to allow patients to return to some 'normality'. Not only will this help with their mental wellbeing, it will allow them to lead as healthy and active life as possible for as long as possible.

There are over 200 types of cancer but the most common cancers are breast, prostate, lung and bowel which account for 53 per cent of all cancers (Cancer Research UK, 2016a). Figure 1.1 identifies the 20 most common cancers according to Cancer Research UK (2016b).

CAUSATIVE FACTORS FOR CANCER

A cancer diagnosis is more likely as one gets older. The peak age at which cancer occurs is age 85+ while half of cancers are diagnosed in people aged 70 or over. However, Cancer Research UK (2016a) has also noted increases in cancers at younger ages too (see Figure 1.2).

Apart from age there are certain lifestyle factors that increase the risk of cancer. The key ones are smoking, poor diet, being overweight and lack of exercise. Cancer Research UK (2016a) estimates that 42 per cent of cancers are preventable. Ensuring a healthy lifestyle significantly reduces the risk of getting cancer (NHS Choices, 2017). In some cases, however, the cause of the cancer is not known.

Interestingly, in my case the type of cancer I developed was not linked to any of the above factors! I was in my fifties, happily married with three grown-up step daughters. I worked as a GP practice manager, a job I loved. I was very fit. I was a keen cyclist and often went on cycling holidays. I also liked walking and went to

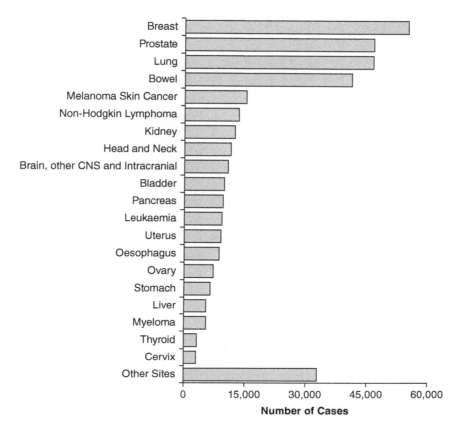

Figure 1.1   Twenty most common cancers in 2014

Source: Reproduced with kind permission of Cancer Research UK

keep fit classes. I had never smoked, drank very little alcohol, ate healthily and had never been overweight. However, one day my life was to change when I began my cancer journey.

GETTING DIAGNOSED: MY EXPERIENCE

In my case it all began one day with a sneeze. One morning as I was about to say goodbye to my husband and head off to work I suddenly gave an almighty sneeze. I immediately said, 'Oh my back!' I thought I'd pulled a muscle as a result of the sneeze. I went to work as usual but over the next few days the pain got worse. Thinking I'd pulled a muscle I decided to have physiotherapy. Initially this seemed to help but then the pain got worse.

I was still going to work but because of the pain I couldn't drive so became reliant on my husband or daughter taking me. I found it impossible to lift things, even a full kettle or my briefcase. I was taking increasing amounts of over the counter

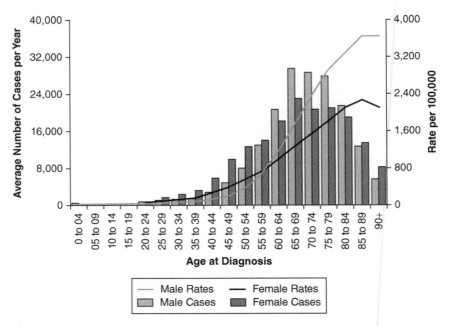

Figure 1.2   All cancers (C00-C97 Excl. C44), average number of new cases per year and age-specific incidence rates per 100,000 population, UK, 2013–2015

Source: Reproduced with kind permission of Cancer Research UK

pain killers. In the end I had to stop them because they caused severe stomach pains. One day I came out of the physiotherapist in tears as the pain was so bad. I had been for early morning appointments and then going straight to work but that day I knew I couldn't cope any more and told my daughter to take me home.

I managed to get an emergency appointment with the registrar at the GP practice. She prescribed stronger pain killers and sent me for a back X-ray. Because of the severe pain I decided to see an orthopaedic consultant privately. I went to the GP practice to collect the referral letter and, if possible, a copy of the X-ray report. The X-ray showed that I had two collapsed vertebrae and that my back was 'highly paretic for a woman of her age' (i.e. I had developed osteoporosis). The GP asked why I was bothering to see a consultant as he'd probably just put me on calcium tablets!

The following day I saw the orthopaedic consultant who measured my height and I was horrified to discover I had lost 2 inches. He realised that I was in considerable pain and said he wanted to admit me in order to carry out tests. The following morning I received a telephone call from the hospital to ask if I could have an MRSA test prior to admission. A couple of days later I was told it was clear and to come to the hospital the following morning.

After admission I had various tests and scans including a radioisotope scan, an MRI scan, X-rays, etc. The consultant orthopaedic surgeon, I realised afterwards, was looking for a tumour but couldn't find anything. He brought in the consultant rheumatologist because of the osteoporosis, and he requested a urine sample to undertake a Bence Jones test, but I did not know the significance of this until later. This is a urine sample test for a protein called Bence Jones (or free light chains), where the body produces antibodies that are incomplete. The presence of any Bence Jones protein in urine suggests an abnormality. These free light chains can cause damage to the kidneys, which is why the presence of this protein is an indicator of myeloma.

I spent a month in hospital. During this time I became quite immobile due to the severe back pain. I was fitted with a back brace, which needed to be put on before I could get out of bed. It took two nurses to get me out of bed each morning and to ease me into it at night. I was unable to shower because of the pain and so during this time was given a shower by one of the nurses. I found the experience of being washed by someone extremely embarrassing although I know for nurses it is an everyday occurrence. This was not helped by the fact that while in the shower another nurse came in to discuss her pay slip and left the door ajar while doing so!

On discharge I had real difficulty going up and down stairs and in dressing. When I had a shower I struggled to lift my hands above my head to wash my hair. I found it hard to get in and out of a chair. One day I tried to open a tin of beans for my lunch and didn't have the strength to use the can opener.

A month after discharge I went to see the consultant rheumatologist. I was doing a little bit at work but was keen to get back to work full time and wanted to know when the treatment for the osteoporosis would allow me to do so. It was then he told me that he'd had the result of the Bence Jones test which showed I had multiple myeloma. I had vaguely heard of myeloma, but knew nothing much about it. My husband had never heard of it. This is not surprising as Myeloma UK estimate that 97 per cent of the population have never heard of myeloma despite it being the second most common form of blood cancer.

The consultant rheumatologist said that I needed to see a haematologist and, as there was a clinic at the hospital that day, he'd ring the haematologist to see if I could be fitted in to the clinic. An hour later I saw the haematologist who said I had light chain myeloma and explained very clearly what it meant.

MULTIPLE MYELOMA

Myeloma, also known as multiple myeloma, is a type of cancer arising from plasma cells. Plasma cells form part of the immune system and are found in the bone marrow. Normal plasma cells produce antibodies to fight infection. In myeloma, abnormal plasma cells release one type of antibody which has no useful function (Manier et al., 2017). Myeloma is different from many other cancers as it does not exist as a lump or tumour; instead abnormal plasma cells multiply and expand within the bone marrow. Myeloma affects multiple places in the body, hence the term multiple myeloma. A large majority of myeloma patients will have IgG or IgA myeloma. This is where the body produces too many of one type of heavy chain antibodies. Free light chain myeloma accounts for about 20 per cent of patients and is where the body produces antibodies that are incomplete – the Bence Jones protein.

One of the most important factors in achieving positive outcomes following a diagnosis of cancer is the speed of obtaining a diagnosis and starting treatment. In the case of myeloma, diagnosis is often quite delayed. This is because in many cases the symptoms, such as fatigue and back pain, are vague and could apply to many illnesses. Lyratzopoulos et al. (2012) identified myeloma as the most difficult of all cancers to diagnose. Indeed 10 per cent of patients die within 60 days of diagnosis (Myeloma UK, 2018). Rapid diagnosis is key to ensuring fewer complications, improved quality of life and better survival outcomes.

The time frame from the initial sneeze to getting a diagnosis of myeloma was about three months. This compares favourably to many patients who are subsequently diagnosed with myeloma as 51 per cent of patients visit their GP at least three times before a diagnosis is confirmed by a haematologist (Lyratzopoulos et al., 2012). As result Myeloma UK (2014) has produced a diagnostic pathway for GPs to assist with speedy diagnosis which suggests 'Think myeloma' if the patient has one or more of the following presentations. Box 1.1 illustrates the common presentations for myeloma.

BOX 1.1   COMMON PRESENTATIONS FOR MYELOMA

- **C**alcium raised or hypercalcaemia – vomiting, nausea, constipation, confusion, bone pain, polyuria
- **R**enal impairment or failure
- **A**naemia – fatigue and shortness of breath
- **B**one lesions, fractures or spinal cord compression – bone pain, particularly non-improving back and/or rib pain, or sudden and/or severe onset of pain, loss of height, or osteoporosis in a man or rapid onset in a woman (Manier et al., 2017).

REACTION TO DIAGNOSIS

In the initial consultation the consultant haematologist told me that myeloma was treatable but not curable. At that stage I realised it was a form of cancer and confess to having had a little cry. The specialist nurse then spent some time reassuring me and giving me more information on myeloma. Later that day I had a bone marrow biopsy. This was carried out to confirm diagnosis and determine the amount of abnormal plasma cells in the bone marrow. A sample of bone marrow is usually taken from the hip bone and examined under the microscope.

I wanted to understand what myeloma was and about the treatments, as my way of coping was to feel I had some control over what was happening. I read the booklet I had been given by the nurse specialist and was fine until I got to the final sentence which read 'three years after diagnosis 50 per cent of patients are alive and well'. My immediate reaction was to worry about the other 50 per cent and which half I would be in.

At first I found it hard to tell people about the diagnosis, especially members of my family. I didn't want to upset people and wasn't sure what their reaction might be. I particularly found it hard to tell my mother. My mother was elderly and getting frail and lived on her own. As she lived a long way away I asked my brother to tell her in person rather than just giving her a telephone call.

I wanted to explore my feelings about getting cancer and found this difficult. Although I wanted to talk about how I felt and what it meant to me I did not want to upset those close to me. It wasn't until a few weeks later that my husband and I had a meaningful conversation about it. Friends who had been visiting had just left and I apologised if I'd not been as chatty as normal but confessed I had felt rather down that day. When I told my husband this it started a conversation about how we both felt.

The diagnosis not only impacted on me. Although my husband had never heard of myeloma he realised from what the consultant haematologist had said that it was serious. He says initially he felt numb and spent the rest of the day in a daze. He went to work the following day but found it hard to concentrate. He also felt angry but he did not know why or who he was angry with – it just seemed so unfair as I had always looked after my health.

TREATMENT EFFECTS

The week after diagnosis the haematologist explained that I was to start chemotherapy and prescribed a combination of drugs on a three-week cycle. This involved taking a chemotherapy tablet, cyclophosphamide, once a week; dexamethasone, a steroid, with a pattern of four days on seven days off; and daily thalidomide.

Ten days after starting the chemotherapy, I suddenly felt terrible and started to shake uncontrollably. According to my daughter my eyes glazed over. I could not face food but went to bed for a few hours and when I got up later felt slightly better. Chemotherapy has a number of side effects although these could be called effects because they were not minor (see Box 1.2).

The following day I had an 'access to work' appointment where they were going to assess what I needed at work to support my back. When I arrived the staff all said I looked terrible and although I had initially planned to stay and do some work I went home after the assessment. Thinking it was simply a reaction to the drugs I contacted the specialist nurse who advised me to come and see the haematologist. I was staggered when the consultant told me I needed to be admitted.

BOX 1.2   COMMON SIDE EFFECTS OF CHEMOTHERAPY

Cyclophosphamide – Risk of infection,* bruising and bleeding,* feeling sick, anaemia,* blood clot risk, sore mouth, hair loss,* constipation,* skin changes, nail changes,* build-up of fluid (oedema)*

Thalidomide – Numb or tingling hands or feet (peripheral neuropathy),* effects on the nervous system, constipation,* skin changes

Dexamethasone – Tummy pain and/or indigestion,* increased appetite, raised blood sugar levels, mood and behaviour changes* (Lorusso et al., 2017)

*Experienced by the author

ADDED COMPLICATIONS

Following my admission to hospital, I was asked to produce a urine sample. Unfortunately, I was unable to do so. This seemed to set off alarm bells. I was catheterised to see if that would help. For some reason the idea of this horrified me and I was very frightened but a lovely nurse said it wouldn't hurt and she'd be very gentle and she was right. Unfortunately, catheterisation made no difference.

The haematologist told me that I would be transferred to the high dependency unit as my kidneys had failed. The haematologist was keen to get me to a specialist centre, and a few days later I was transferred to the high dependency unit at a renal centre. This transfer took place late at night and I remember the junior doctor and the night nurse asking me lots of questions. When I asked what time it was when the doctor had finished she said it was 3.00 a.m.! The nurse had a checklist and one of the questions was 'How positive do you feel about life?' While I'm sure being aware of the patient's psychological state is important it didn't seem the best time or way to ask.

During my time in the specialist renal unit I had a kidney biopsy and was told I had 'cast nephropathy' which meant that my kidneys had failed and they considered the damage to be permanent. Myeloma cast nephropathy is the formation of plugs (urinary casts) in the renal tubules from free immunoglobulin light chains leading to renal failure in the context of multiple myeloma (Demaria et al., 2017).

REFLECTIONS ON HOSPITAL EXPERIENCE

I was on haemodialysis three days a week and found the dialysis quite exhausting. My time in hospital as a patient was not always a positive experience. This was a really difficult time for me. I had a lot of oedema in my legs partly as a result of all the fluid that had been pumped into me. I was told to keep my legs elevated when sitting in a chair but found this really hard as it was extremely painful for my back.

The bed rest on the hospital bed was broken and did not work and I could not sit up in bed without this support. This meant it was incredibly difficult to get comfortable and the only way was to lie down. I was even lying down when meals were brought. These were placed on a bed table above me and I could not really see the plate and what I was eating. It was not easy to eat without making a mess in such a position.

Another particular problem I had was the loss of dexterity in my fingers. I could not hold a pen. I found this inability to write one of the most disturbing aspects as I was someone who would normally write things down or make lists. I was never told why this occurred but subsequently discovered another myeloma patient who had a similar problem.

As it was a teaching hospital the consultants came round with their 'entourage'. I recall a consultant haematologist coming in along with his entire team while my husband was visiting. While they were there the renal consultant also came in and my husband counted 17 people in my side room. I told the specialist haematology nurse that I had found it rather inhibiting and overwhelming and I'm glad to say that it was never repeated.

I was initially confined to the room because I was on oxygen. Once this was removed I found, because of the oedema and general weakness, that I had lost my mobility. Physiotherapy helped but I remember that the first walk I took with the physiotherapist was only about 12 steps from the bed and was quite exhausting. However, as I gained more strength, I was able to practise each day and even get outside of the ward. It was great to see the 'real world' again, even if it wasn't beautiful countryside.

While in hospital the same junior doctor who admitted me noticed that the blood results implied that I had some kidney function returning. They decided not to give me dialysis but monitor the situation and reassured me that if necessary I would be given dialysis. My kidney function continued to improve and when I was discharged a month after the original admission I was not on dialysis. This was the best news I'd had since I first became ill.

CONTINUING TREATMENT

Having just spent a month in hospital, I was only back home a week when I started to feel poorly again. I had an infection and diarrhoea. This had previously occurred when I was in the specialist renal unit so I contacted my GP to see if I could be prescribed the same antibiotics. She in turn contacted the haematologist for advice and then came to see me and told me if I got any worse to go to the haematology ward. Unfortunately, I did get worse and I had a further admission.

This admission resulted in another month in hospital. Yet again I had various infusions. As a result the oedema got worse and I had 'elephant legs' and even oedema on my torso. I was in a side room and liked the privacy. I even had the luxury of an en-suite bathroom but the high lip to the shower cubicle meant I simply couldn't use it. This time the nurses gave me a bath using a hoist and while

I was less worried about being naked I found the hoist quite scary. However, the bath itself was glorious.

During my stay I completely lost my appetite and initially couldn't face food and was losing weight. As a result, on the advice of the dietician, a nurse inserted a nasogastric tube to feed me that way. As with the initial urinary catheter this really freaked me out and I hated the thought of someone inserting a tube up my nose and down my throat. They gave me a sedative first as I was so agitated about it and I requested that someone might hold my hand. I found that my way of coping with anything unpleasant was to close my eyes so I couldn't see what they were doing and to have someone hold my hand. Just as a child might clutch a toy or blanket, this was my comforter. The nurse who inserted the tube was lovely and very calming and she brought a colleague with her who held my hand. I was told I was the perfect patient and swallowed hard when they told me to.

The experience of having a nasogastric tube was very unpleasant. I hated being fed this way and found I felt constantly bloated and full. One evening, as I had started to eat again, I refused to have any more feed. The following day the dietician came to see me as she had heard of my refusal and said that provided I ate the meals and snacks I wouldn't have to be fed by the nasogastric tube. She ordered extra snacks for me alongside build-up type drinks. The latter were supposed to taste of fruit juice. I found them disgusting but managed to sip them gradually during the day.

One weekend they allowed me to go home overnight but I had to come back in the morning for a heparin injection. It was lovely being at home and my husband cooked a meal. I don't remember exactly what it was, but do recall that it included some new potatoes with butter which tasted wonderful after being used to hospital mashed potatoes. During the night I got up to go to the toilet and then could not get up from the toilet seat. It took 45 minutes to get me up and this upset me. I told the nurse when I went to the hospital for the injection and she gave me a raised toilet seat to take home. The frame went over the toilet and this made all the difference. Four weeks after my initial admission I was back home and started to make steady improvements in mobility.

Because of the added complication of the kidney problem the chemotherapy dosage was reduced. Although initially I was told that I would have six cycles of treatment, in the event I had nine. The intention was to reduce the myeloma so that I could then undergo a stem cell transplant. A stem cell transplant, sometimes called a bone marrow transplant, aims to give patients healthy stem cells which then produce normal blood cells. There are two types of stem cell transplant: autologous, or autograft, using the patient's own stem cells and allogenic, or allograft, which uses donor stem cells and is a higher-risk procedure.

STEM CELL TRANSPLANT

Almost a year after my sneeze I had a stem cell transplant. My siblings had been tested but unfortunately they were not a match. Using donor stem cells gives the best chance of a 'cure' although it carries greater risks. In my case I had an autologous stem cell transplant. This is the most common type of transplant with myeloma patients.

In preparation for the stem cell transplant, I had intravenous chemotherapy to kill off all the remaining myeloma cells and then hormone injections to increase the growth of my own stem cells. Unfortunately I got a urinary infection and so, rather than having the injections at home, I was once again in hospital. My stem cell level was monitored daily. It took a while for the stem cells to come up to the necessary level.

When I had started to grow my own stem cells, the excess cells were taken out of my blood by simply removing some of my blood via a femoral line. This was put through a centrifuge; the stem cells were separated out before returning the blood. Normally the aim is to get sufficient stem cells for two transplants but in my case they just got sufficient stem cells for one transplant.

About a month later I had yet more chemotherapy before they returned the stem cells to me. There were two short infusions of stem cells and immediately after the first one I was sick. The next few weeks were the worst of my life. I developed rampant diarrhoea, so much so that I had to wear incontinence pads like large nappies and despite this I still managed to soil myself. If I tried to eat anything I was promptly sick, despite the fact that I was given anti-sickness tablets. I even found it hard to swallow tablets without retching. Wherever possible the staff used a Hickman line, an intravenous catheter which was inserted in the jugular vein, to give me all my medications. I also had mouth ulcers and a dry mouth and I found myself sucking lots of ice pops as I found this soothing on the mouth and easier than drinking fluids.

Although I had been told in advance about the risks and indeed the side effects of the transplant I think it was worse than I imagined. Prior to the treatment I had started to feel a bit better and the treatment itself caused me to feel much worse. In cancer treatment patients often suffer from what is referred to as iatrogenesis where the medication itself causes the illness and this was true in my case.

THE IMPLICATIONS OF THE CANCER EXPERIENCE: IMPACT ON THE FAMILY

A cancer diagnosis does not just affect the patient but also other members of the family. As mentioned earlier, initially my husband felt numb and then angry but overall he felt worried. This level of anxiety increased when I went into renal failure. During my first year of illness I spent 17 weeks in hospital, which put a strain on him trying to fit in visiting, running a home and work. In the end he decided that it was work that had to go.

He managed to take early retirement but because he was only 56 his pension was reduced. Fortunately we still had sufficient income to have no real financial worries, but for many people a cancer diagnosis brings with it financial concerns too.

Even when I was at home, suddenly he had turned from being a partner into a full-time carer. Although we had always shared jobs around the house he now had to do everything as most of that first year I was incapable of doing household tasks.

He also felt he needed time for himself yet was reluctant to leave me for long. Initially he came with me to the cancer care centre and had a couple of counselling sessions which he found helpful. He also had aromatherapy which, much to his surprise, he found very relaxing. He continued to go cycling with friends on a Sunday morning. This gave him the opportunity to talk to people and really helped clear his mind.

POST-TRANSPLANT

After another four-week spell in hospital I was discharged and started to make slow but steady progress. I started to be able to eat again, having lost a lot of weight and my appetite.

I was able to go on holiday about five months after the transplant. Our holidays used to be quite active but this was no longer feasible. We chose to go on a cruise because I thought it would give us a chance to see lots of places and my husband could use the facilities on the ship. We had always been keen travellers and when I initially became ill had to cancel a touring holiday to Morocco which included trips into the High Atlas Mountains. It was our first holiday in two years. I used the wheelchair, which limited what we could do, but it was lovely to get a break and good for my husband too.

Both before and after the stem cell transplant I would have regular blood transfusions when my full blood count or haemoglobin became very low. After the transplant the haematologist referred me back to the renal unit as he diagnosed renal anaemia. I started having EPO (or erythropoietin) injections which increases the red blood cells. I'd always hated needles, and although I'd had numerous blood tests because of the nature of the cancer I was not very happy with the idea of injecting myself. However, after some training with the nurse at the GP practice I managed it myself. EPO has made a huge difference as I have had no more blood transfusions and have more energy as a result of the increase in my haemoglobin or full blood count.

After the transplant I attended the haematology clinic regularly and it became routine. One day my husband had to take my daughter to get her car repaired and so for the first time I was at clinic on my own. That day I was told that I had high calcium and they thought the myeloma was coming back. I was told I was to be admitted and that I needed another bone marrow biopsy. Until then I'd remained fairly positive but the thought that after less than a year since the transplant the myeloma had come back was very upsetting and I got quite low. Fortunately the bone marrow biopsy was clear and after a few days I was allowed home.

The next hiccup was the reverse, I had low calcium. I had regular monthly infusions of pamidronate which was a drug prescribed to protect the bones. I usually organised it so that I had bloods taken followed by the infusion before I saw the consultant in the clinic. One day while attached to the drip, a nurse said that the pathology department had been in contact with the consultant because my calcium levels were very low and they needed to stop the infusion immediately as this would lower it still further.

I subsequently saw the consultant haematologist but felt fine and went home as normal. That evening I had some friends round as we were in a book club and I was going to comment on the book and realised that I couldn't speak properly. My speech was slurred and I had difficulty forming words. It was quite scary. We abandoned book club and I went to the A&E at the hospital where I was admitted and given infusions of calcium, which resolved the problem although I don't think they knew what caused the level to drop.

I still attended the renal clinic but not very frequently. About a year after the stem cell transplant at a routine appointment they noted a large amount of protein in the urine and told me that I needed another kidney biopsy. I had the biopsy and came back to clinic a month later for the results. I was told it showed that my kidneys were failing and that I'd need dialysis within the year.

RENAL FAILURE

The day that I was told that I'd need to go back on dialysis I felt understandably low. I worried that my life would never be the same. My husband and I had booked a holiday to Switzerland for the following month. We were told it was fine to go but by the end of the holiday I started to feel generally unwell, very tired and had lost my appetite.

A specialist renal nurse visited me at home and patiently and carefully talked about the different options for dialysis. I chose to have peritoneal dialysis (PD). PD is the process of removing excess fluid and metabolic by-products from the body by circulating dialysis solution through the peritoneal cavity using a peritoneal catheter (an exchange). Haemodialysis involves diverting blood into an external machine, where it's filtered before being returned to the body. Because of the underlying myeloma which had affected the kidneys and caused them to fail I would not be placed on the transplant list so would be on dialysis for the rest of my life. My kidneys deteriorated faster than anticipated and three months after the biopsy I started dialysis. Table 1.1 demonstrates the differences between the two types of dialysis.

Table 1.1   Haemodialysis vs peritoneal dialysis (Stadlbauer et al., 2017)

	Haemodialysis	Peritoneal dialysis
Access	Via a fistula in the arm	Via a Tenckhoff catheter in the stomach
Location	Renal unit	Home
Frequency	3 times a week	Daily
Diet	Very restricted	Some restrictions
Storage	None	Large quantities of fluid

Source: Reproduced with permission under the terms of the Creative Commons CC BY licence.

I found the initial regime of continuous ambulatory peritoneal dialysis (CAPD), whereby I did four exchanges a day, very disruptive to my life. It was difficult to go out anywhere as I was always anxious to get back home for an exchange. After about 12 weeks I transferred to using a machine which basically did the same thing but completed a number of exchanges while I was sleeping. I received training in using the machine at home and remember my first night on it was on a Christmas Eve which gave me a lovely free Christmas Day that year.

THE SUPPORTING ROLE OF THE NURSE

At the very start of my cancer journey I was fortunate in having an excellent hae-matology nurse. On the very first day that I was given the diagnosis she spent time reassuring me. I found her so approachable and she supported not only me but members of my family too.

The haematology nurse specialist put me in touch with another patient with myeloma which was very helpful as I had never met anyone with myeloma. She was keen to start a support group for patients with myeloma and persuaded us both to start a group which has now been running for ten years. I found that being able to share experiences with other myeloma patients a great help. I now feel able to help others in this respect too. Helping to run the support group also gave me a sense of purpose and an opportunity to use my organisational skills.

I also found that little things made a big difference to me. For example, one of the early scans involved going to another hospital accompanied by a nurse. She was sub-sequently on another ward but came to see me before her shift started to see how I was. Another nurse noticed that the skin on my feet was peeling off and got some cream and massaged it in. Others held my hand when I had procedures that worried me. They praised me for being brave when I had certain procedures such as inserting a femoral line. They chatted to me while doing tasks such as changing the bed. All of these helped build relationships and made me feel a person, not just a patient.

SUPPORTIVE INTERVENTIONS

Not long after being diagnosed I heard of a cancer support centre and went there for a few weeks. They provided counselling for me and my husband and also com-plementary therapies, both of which helped me to become more positive.

While I was in hospital for the stem cell transplant I had reflexology which I found very relaxing. I have continued to have complementary therapy post treat-ment as I have found it has helped with my general wellbeing and recovery.

I have also been extremely fortunate to have a supportive family and a wide circle of friends who came to visit me both in the hospital and at home. I found that this acted as distraction therapy and even found that I did not feel the same need for painkillers when I was otherwise occupied. I also found that friends would take me shopping in my wheelchair and this was not only good for me but gave my husband a break too.

LIVING WITH MYELOMA

Having myeloma and the effects of the renal failure has had a significant impact on my life. Firstly I took ill health retirement at the age of 54 and my husband took early retirement to look after me. Neither of us had intended to retire that early and of course this had an impact on our income although fortunately our reduced income was still sufficient for our needs.

The year following that fateful sneeze I spent 17 weeks in hospital which was very disruptive to family life. I was not able to help run the home as I normally would and was very reliant on my husband.

Prior to taking ill we had both been keen cyclists and walkers, and holidays tended to involve one or both activities. I could no longer cycle and indeed was for some considerable time using a wheelchair. I was not able to drive for quite some time because of both general weakness and the inability to turn my head to look behind. I therefore lost a lot of independence and became dependent on my husband or friends to take me anywhere.

I also found the impact on my body image initially very difficult. The chemotherapy led to hair loss and although I did get a wig I found it itchy and uncomfortable. I had lost over 5 inches in height, which not only changed my body shape so none of my clothes fitted I felt tiny next to my 6 foot 2 inch husband. I had also developed a curvature as a result of the osteoporosis. Finally, I was very conscious of the permanent catheter in my stomach. One of the disadvantages of peritoneal dialysis is that it causes constipation. I started taking two laxatives per day but quickly realised that this was insufficient. I increased this to eight tablets a day, and despite this initially I sometimes still had to take additional laxatives. Fortunately, as I have become more active, this is now better controlled.

Another problem with PD dialysis is the storage of all the fluid and peripheral equipment. I receive a monthly delivery of supplies. After a delivery I can have nearly 60 boxes of fluid and other supplies to store weighing over half a ton. This means one spare bedroom is virtually a storeroom. All of the effects of the illness and the treatment have, at times, caused significant changes to my life.

The specialist haematology nurse and the specialist renal nurse were extremely supportive during my treatment and subsequently. They were always there for advice and initially I called on them a lot, but as time went on I felt able to manage most situations myself. They encouraged me to live life to the full. For example, the nurses encouraged me to go on holiday despite the dialysis.

TAKING BACK CONTROL

As mentioned earlier, I wanted to be able to know about the illness as I wanted to take some control over my life. As I started to feel stronger I asked my GP to refer me to 'exercise on prescription'. Initially I was given a programme of gym exercises which was reviewed at regular intervals. I was also given information about local walks and it was suggested that I took up tai chi. After a year I gave up the gym as I found it boring but carried on with tai chi and walking and also started to do short bike rides and, more recently, going to Zumba. I found the exercise made me stronger physically and also improved my mood. It also helped with the constipation that is associated with the dialysis.

Macmillan (2013) proposes education and support events are held post treatment to encourage people to lead a healthy lifestyle. These were not available after my treatment but instinctively I continued to have a healthy diet, albeit with restrictions because of the PD. I followed the dietician's advice very strictly and as a result my dialysis has been well controlled.

I still manage to go on holiday despite the dialysis as the equipment I need is sent out to the hotel in advance. While I may not be able to go to exotic locations because of back-up facilities and infection risks I have travelled to nine European countries and all nations of the UK since I started on dialysis.

I have found that keeping up with exercise and having a wide circle of friends and active social life has kept me positive. I know that myeloma is a remitting cancer and is likely to come back at some stage but I do not worry about it on a daily basis but keep planning ahead.

CONCLUSION

The high incidence of cancer means that there is a 1 in 2 risk of developing cancer during one's lifetime. Many cancers are preventable or at least one can significantly reduce the risk of getting cancer by having a healthy lifestyle. For others such as myself there is as yet no known cause of my type of cancer.

Many cancer treatments cause significant side effects. In my case these included hair loss, nausea, diarrhoea, constipation, oedema, neuropathy and reduced mobility. Reflecting on my personal experiences, I was impressed by the small acts of kindness nurses carried out to help me cope with the treatments and their side effects – for example, the nurse who noticed my feet were in a terrible condition and massaged them with cream, and the nurses who held my hand when having worrying procedures such as kidney biopsy or nasogastric tube insertion.

I also experienced positive experiences of complementary medicine which helped relieve the symptoms and lifted my mood.

A cancer diagnosis not only impacts on the patient but also on those closest to them and can lead to major changes in the lives of patients and family members. After treatment the patient may have to cope with a new 'norm', which in my case meant coming to terms with loss of height, curvature and most significantly renal failure leading to the need for dialysis.

After treatment has been completed keeping socially and physically active can also help maintain a positive attitude as well as improve outcomes. Nurses can help support patients to live an active life when treatment has been completed and be accessible when needed.

Treatments for cancer are improving all the time so that more and more people are surviving cancer. However, cancer can leave people with having to cope with the after-effects of treatment and/or the cancer itself. The challenge for professionals is to empower patients to live a healthy and active life post treatment and take back control.

REFERENCES

Cancer Research UK (2016a) *Cancer Risk Statistics*. Available at www.cancerresearchuk.org/health-professional/cancer-statistics/risk, accessed December 2016.

Cancer Research UK (2016b) *Cancer Incidence for Common Cancers*. Available at www.cancerresearchuk.org/health-professional/cancer-statistics/incidence/common-cancers-compared#heading-Zero, accessed December 2016.

Demaria, M., O'Leary, M.N., Chang, J., Shao, L. et al. (2017) 'Cellular senescence promotes adverse effects of chemotherapy and cancer relapse.' *Cancer Discovery*, 7 (2): 165–76.

Glaser, A.W., Fraser, L.K., Corner, J., Feltbower, R. et al. (2013) 'Patient reported outcomes of cancer survivors in England 1–5 years after diagnosis: a cross-sectional survey.' *BMJ Open*, 8 August 2013.

Lorusso, D., Bria, E., Costantini, A., Di Maio, M., Rosti, G. and Mancuso, A. (2017) 'Patients' perception of chemotherapy side effects: expectations, doctor–patient communication and impact on quality of life – an Italian survey.' *European Journal of Cancer Care*, 26 (2): e12618.

Lyratzopoulos, G., Neal, R.D., Barbiere, J.M., Ripin, G.P. and Abel, G.A. (2012) 'Variation in number of general practitioner consultations before hospital referral for cancer: findings from the 2010 National Cancer Patient Experience Survey in England.' *Lancet Oncol*, 13 (4): 353–65.

Macmillan (2013) *The Recovery Package*, MAC15514.

Manier, S., Salem, K.Z., Park, J., Landa, D.A., Getz, G. and Ghobrial, I.M. (2017) 'Genomic complexity of multiple myeloma and its clinical implications.' *Nature Reviews in Clinical Oncology*, 14: 100–13.

Morgan, M.A. (2009) 'Cancer survivorship: history, quality-of-life issues, and the evolving multidisciplinary approach to cancer survivorship care plans.' *Oncology Nursing Forum*, 36 (4): 429–36.

Myeloma UK (2018) *Myeloma Diagnosis Pathway*. Available at https://academy.myeloma.org.uk/wp-content/uploads/sites/2/2015/04/Myeloma-UK-Myeloma-Diagnosis-Pathway.pdf, accessed June 2018.

NHS Choices (2017) *Cancer*. Available at www.nhs.uk/conditions/cancer/Pages/Introduction.aspx, accessed December 2016.

Stadlbauer, V., Horvath, A., Ribitsch, W., Schmerböck, B. et al. (2017) 'Structural and functional differences in gut microbiome composition in patients undergoing haemodialysis or peritoneal dialysis.' *Scientific Reports*, 7. doi:10.1038/s41598-017-15650-9. University Journal of Pre and Para Clinical Sciences ISSN 2455–2879 Volume 3 Issue 1.203.199.194.74

2

PALLIATIVE CARE FOR PEOPLE WITH END STAGE PULMONARY DISEASE

JOSEPHINE POPLE

LEARNING OUTCOMES

- Gain a clearer understanding of how to recognise the stages of ESPD
- Develop an awareness of how healthcare professionals can use supportive management to ease the physical, psychological and social aspects of the disease
- Outline the nursing challenges associated with providing palliative and end of life care specific to end stage pulmonary disease (ESPD)

INTRODUCTION

End stage pulmonary disease (ESPD) is a complex and variable illness characterised by long-term deterioration of the respiratory system, leading to a diminished ability to breathe. This chapter extends the commonly used term chronic obstructive pulmonary disease (COPD) to the more contemporary term 'end stage pulmonary disease' (ESPD). An overview of the pathophysiology of chronic lung disease is provided in order to demonstrate how chronic respiratory disease can develop, with the patient becoming increasingly breathless and requiring greater levels of intervention. The chapter highlights the transition from the need for acute intervention to a situation where the patient requires palliative care, which quite soon becomes end of life care. To highlight the complexity and the changes in a patient's condition the chapter centres on two key case studies (Kenneth and Edith) that enable the reader to focus on the patient's experience and consider the debilitating impact of ESPD on the patient. The case studies also help to draw together the key factors in providing optimal palliative care and eventually end of life care.

OVERVIEW OF PULMONARY DISEASE

The rising prevalence of non-malignant pulmonary disease reached over 1.5 million people in the UK by 2013, with more people diagnosed in deprived areas; 5.3 per cent of all deaths were attributed to COPD alone (BLF, 2016). The main cause was exposure to cigarette smoke. However, a small proportion (1%) of sufferers were deficient in alpha-1 antitrypsin, a protein involved in promoting healthy lung tissue. Fewer than half of smokers develop COPD, suggesting a genetic involvement (Rennard and Vestbo, 2006). There is less detailed statistical data regarding the prevalence of other progressive lung diseases. However, a national report from 2012 showed that a total of 5,292 people died from idiopathic pulmonary fibrosis (BLF, 2017), while the prevalence of asbestosis is relatively smaller, with 467 deaths due to the illness in 2015 (HSE, 2017). ESPD encompasses a range of lung conditions, therefore the patient's illness trajectory varies greatly.

People with lung disease can begin their illness with one lung problem such as bronchitis related to their lifestyle or environment and thereafter develop other lung conditions which may co-exist with the primary disease. Box 2.1 lists the types of chronic lung conditions that can lead to end stage pulmonary disease. As the conditions progress over time, lung function deteriorates and the diseases advance to what is known as 'end stage' pulmonary disease. Despite lung cancer and mesothelioma often developing into an end stage pulmonary disease, they will not be discussed in this section as they are malignant illnesses. Note that asthma is not classified as an 'end stage' disease as it does not demonstrate the same progression as the other conditions. However, a severe attack can be fatal (Arshad and Babu, 2008).

BOX 2.1   TYPES OF CHRONIC LUNG CONDITIONS THAT CAN LEAD TO END STAGE PULMONARY DISEASE

- Asbestosis
- Asthma (this does not lead to ESPD)
- Bronchiectasis
- COPD
- Cystic fibrosis
- Lung cancer
- Mesothelioma
- Pulmonary fibrosis
- Pulmonary sarcoidosis

SIGNS AND SYMPTOMS OF ESPD

The extent to which people experience ESPD varies depending on the type and amount of damage to the lung. The literature and statistical data often focus on the term COPD, as this is the most prevalent subtype of ESPD (Snell et al., 2016). Therefore, the most common clinical presentation of patients with ESPD requiring admission to acute care is a chest infection referred to as an infective exacerbation. Typical symptoms include breathlessness (dyspnoea), productive cough, wheezing, chest tightness and fever (Currie and Chetty, 2011). Clinical indicators specific to other subtypes of ESPD include finger clubbing and a non-productive cough in pulmonary fibrosis (Nakamura and Suda, 2015). Sarcoidosis can involve red lumps on the skin, lymphadenopathy, and painful joints in addition to breathlessness (Mitchell et al., 2012).

As the disease advances, lung function deteriorates, which can result in acute-on-chronic respiratory failure. There are two types of respiratory failure: type I, which is defined as hypoxaemia (low oxygen levels), and type II, hypoxaemia with hypercapnia (high carbon dioxide levels) (Gnanapandithan and Agarwal, 2012). Advanced COPD in particular is commonly associated with type II failure, and complications arise with oxygen administration; too much oxygen can induce dangerous levels of carbon dioxide retention (Abdo and Heunks, 2012). Effros and Swenson (2016) describe the three main mechanisms: hypoventilation of the alveoli, a 'mismatch' of the ventilation and perfusion of the alveoli, and what's known as the 'Haldane effect', which involves the red blood cells' affinity for oxygen and carbon dioxide. This can lead to serious issues such as drowsiness and confusion, which if left untreated can be fatal (Abdo and Heunks, 2012). For those with ESPD, ethical decisions have to be made regarding the level of ventilation appropriate for the patient, an issue that will be explored later in the chapter and in more detail in Chapter 10.

ESPD ASSESSMENT

ESPD assessment should take into account the type and severity of symptoms, previous exacerbations, comorbidities, as well as the degree of airflow limitation. Spirometry results are useful for clinicians to diagnose and monitor, and have been found to be independently associated with subjective experience of breathlessness (Leivseth et al., 2012). The Medical Research Council (MRC) Dyspnoea Scale (see Table 2.1) is often used to ascertain the level of disability present.

Table 2.1   Medical Research Council Dyspnoea Scale

Grade	Degree of breathlessness related to activities
1	Not troubled by breathlessness except on strenuous exercise
2	Short of breath when hurrying or walking up a slight hill
3	Walks slower than contemporaries on the level, stops after a mile or so, or stops after 15 minutes when walking at own pace
4	Stops for breath after walking about 100 metres or after a few minutes on level ground
5	Too breathless to leave the house, or breathless when dressing

Source: Adapted from Stenton (2008)

Case study 2.1 illustrates the impact that breathlessness can have on a person's daily life.

CASE STUDY 2.1   KENNETH

Kenneth suffered from idiopathic pulmonary fibrosis (IPF) and had been struggling with his breathing for the past three years. He was provided with home oxygen via a mask to help his breathing. Over time, however, his breathing deteriorated to the point where he found it difficult to get to the kitchen to make a cup of tea, despite using home oxygen. The walk made him feel exhausted and even the kettle felt heavier, like he had just run a 100m sprint. Despite this, Kenneth wanted to stay mobile and practise the gentle sitting exercises he learned in pulmonary rehabilitation. Kenneth had carers who came in the morning to help him get washed and dressed, which he felt was very helpful. He was also seen by a specialist respiratory nurse, who monitored his condition and provided psychological support for him and his wife Doreen. Despite suffering from a progressive illness, Kenneth was determined to remain positive, and had recently taken to using online forums to share his story and support others with the condition.

This brief case study demonstrates how ESPD can have a profoundly limiting effect on a person's life. However, each individual manages their particular condition and symptoms in different ways; the person's social support often plays a big part in maintaining their psychological wellbeing.

The diagnosis of end stage pulmonary disease should involve a holistic assessment centred on the individual's condition. In addition to the MRC Dyspnoea Scale (see Table 2.1), other tests can be used to assess the severity of the varying illnesses. For example, some argue the six-minute walk test (measuring distance and oxygen saturations) to be a reliable indicator of increased mortality in idiopathic pulmonary fibrosis (Nathan et al., 2015). However, national UK guidelines stress that prognosis should be based on clinical lung function tests (NICE, 2017). While in patients with cystic fibrosis, factors such as low body mass index, number and exacerbations, and the colonisation of particular bacteria can indicate poor survival rates (Aaron et al., 2015).

COMMON PATIENT EXPERIENCES

BREATHLESSNESS

Breathlessness (dyspnoea) is the predominant symptom of ESPD. Initially exertional, it progresses to affect daily activities and eventually is present at rest. The average person takes over 20,000 breaths a day; for those with ESPD, the effort becomes exhausting, leading to feelings of suffocation. Coughing and increased mucus production develops in reaction to bronchial inflammation.

The person's chest may feel tight as the bronchi contract; in some cases there is an audible wheeze (Vestbo, 2010). Many find that positional changes ease breathlessness (see Figure 2.1). Leaning forward onto the elbows in a 'tripod' position and using the support of pillows often helps, whereas lying flat can aggravate breathlessness. Many end up breathing using accessory respiratory muscles, making them feel like they are unable to rest. Multi-posture adjustable beds can be useful to support the patient in hospital and at home if available.

The assessment of patients with ESPD takes place in three stages: 1. Assess; 2. Care; and 3. Evaluate. Figure 2.2 illustrates the assessment stages of the breathless patient followed by the appropriate care which includes addressing the psychological effects of breathlessness. The experience of acute breathlessness can evoke powerful levels of anxiety which are difficult to manage. Patients in such conditions should not be left unaccompanied. Nurses should use a range of communication skills to attempt to reassure the patient that the situation will ease, such as holding their hand or placing a hand on their back. Encouraging deep breathing, use of the oxygen and methods to distract and help induce relaxation can all be effective. If for any reason the situation is getting out of hand, call for senior help. Care interventions should be based on what the individual patient feels will help their breathlessness, as well as their situation.

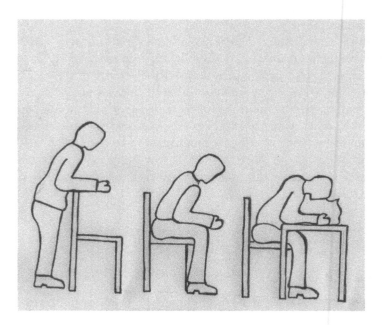

Figure 2.1   Positions to ease breathlessness

Source: Original drawing by Betty Dewey

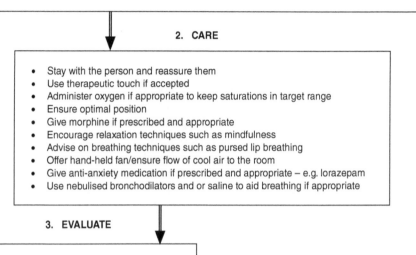

1. ASSESS

- **Check their oxygen saturation level and respiration rate** – They should have a target saturation range, commonly 88-92%
- **Assess the person's skin colour** – A blue or grey can indicate a lack of oxygen and/or infection
- **Are they using accessory muscles?** – This indicates laboured breathing and is exhausting for the patient
- **Assess their position** (see fig 2.1)
- **Are they able to complete full sentences?** – If not, breathlessness is severe and requires immediate intervention
- **Are they using their nose, mouth or both to breath?**
- **Are they using oxygen?**
- **Are there any added sounds to their breathing?** – e.g. wheeze, audible mucus present
- **Do they appear anxious as well as breathless?**
- **Is there visible peripheral or central cyanosis?** – A blue tinge to the skin indicates a lack of oxygen

2. CARE

- Stay with the person and reassure them
- Use therapeutic touch if accepted
- Administer oxygen if appropriate to keep saturations in target range
- Ensure optimal position
- Give morphine if prescribed and appropriate
- Encourage relaxation techniques such as mindfulness
- Advise on breathing techniques such as pursed lip breathing
- Offer hand-held fan/ensure flow of cool air to the room
- Give anti-anxiety medication if prescribed and appropriate – e.g. lorazepam
- Use nebulised bronchodilators and or saline to aid breathing if appropriate

3. EVALUATE

- Evaluate care and reassess regularly
- Escalate to senior colleagues if necessary

Figure 2.2   Taking care of the breathless patient

BOX 2.2   EFFECTS OF BREATHLESSNESS ON ACTIVITIES OF DAILY LIVING (ADL)

- Difficulty talking and maintaining conversation – severe breathlessness may leave the person unable to speak
- Poor sleep – breathlessness can often necessitate the person having their upper body supported (with pillows). Acute episodes of breathlessness can frequently disturb sleep (paroxysmal nocturnal dyspnoea)

(Continued)

(Continued)

- The effort of washing and dressing becomes difficult due to fatigue and breathlessness
- Mobilising becomes more challenging as breathlessness dominates and the body becomes deconditioned
- Eating due to breathlessness can be problematic; valuable body weight can be lost
- Physical intimacy may become difficult to maintain, which can put pressure on relationships
- Hobbies and social activities are affected as the person may struggle to breathe during normal activities; concentrating on something else (e.g. a film) can be hard as anxiety sets in

N.B. If two or more of the criteria are met it indicates severe decline, which triggers palliative care planning (Thomas et al., 2016).

Breathlessness has a profound effect on ADL. Initially, reduced exercise tolerance restricts hill/stair climbing, progressing to limited mobility and ultimately the individual becoming housebound (see Box 2.2). As breathlessness intensifies, the person becomes more socially isolated; there is a global negative impact on the person's work, social and financial spheres of life. This is exacerbated by frequent hospitalisations and increasing physical dependence (Gardiner et al., 2010). Issues then arise with more fundamental aspects of life as breathlessness on rest develops. This contributes to an overall feeling of fatigue and weakness, which is worsened by the increasing effort of breathing itself. Some of the debilitating impact of breathlessness is illustrated in Case study 2.2.

CASE STUDY 2.2   EDITH

Edith was a 70-year-old woman with severe COPD and bronchiectasis. She lived in a two-storey house with her husband Michael and son John who had a learning disability. Michael worked full time while Edith cared for John. Edith had a history of anxiety, right-sided heart failure, and suffered a stroke two years ago, which left her with mild right-sided weakness. She had smoked for around 50 years and still had a cigarette occasionally. Her current medications included inhalers and nebulisers, as well as long-term prophylactic antibiotics, and a yearly flu jab. She took steroids when needed for exacerbations.

Recently, Edith's breathlessness worsened. She was now breathless at rest and found it a struggle to move around the house. She lived downstairs and slept on the sofa with several pillows. She used a commode, and a walking stick for short distances. However, she began feeling increasingly weak and very fatigued. In appearance, she looked hunched over, with fast, shallow breaths. She had lost weight over the past few months (her BMI was 17) and was being encouraged with supplement drinks. The living room was cluttered, with the TV on for background noise; Edith said that she could not concentrate on it any more. She also used to knit but lost patience with it. Social isolation was noticeable; Edith fondly remembered working behind the bar in local pubs, however, she was now embarrassed to leave the house in case someone recognised her. She had ambulatory oxygen (1L via nasal cannula), but resented it and felt that it was a burden.

Her main issue was breathlessness, using an understatement of 'It gets on my nerves'. It is obvious she felt very frustrated and fed up. She wished that 'something had been done earlier' before reaching this stage, and appeared exhausted with the constant mental and physical struggle to manage her breathing. Fresh air helped and she had a hand-held fan that she sometimes used. The community respiratory nurses encouraged her to use the breathing technique they showed her, breathing in through her nose and out through her mouth to help relaxation. They also prescribed a low dose of Oramorph (liquid morphine) to ease the breathlessness; however, Edith was reluctant to use it due to a fear of side effects and becoming dependent. Her overall mood was low and she was upset about her deterioration. There was some underlying anxiety, but she was stoical, perhaps due to her caring responsibilities for John.

Edith was under the care of the community COPD team, who were managing her symptoms at home and aiming to minimise the need for hospital admissions. She also had the support of her GP as well as the respiratory consultant, and recently was seen by a Macmillan nurse, although she declined social care for the time being. Despite this, she felt that no one was helping her as her breathing was becoming more difficult. Edith had some insight into her situation, commenting on how she 'lived in this one room'. However, there had not been any end of life care discussions, a community Do not attempt resuscitation (DNAR) order, or advance care plan (ACP) in place. This was because Edith was finding her situation overwhelming, and was not ready to acknowledge or discuss such difficult topics. She had missed several appointments for spirometry testing to assess the severity of her COPD, which may also have been due to avoidance. Guilt can play a big part in ESPD especially when the patient is a smoker. Edith's respiratory doctor mentioned how her previous factory job may have contributed to her condition, which she says made her feel better about herself.

REFLECTIVE EXERCISE 2.1   EDITH CASE STUDY

1. To what extent does Edith fulfil the criteria for ESPD according to the Gold Standards Framework Prognostic Indicator Guidance (see Box 2.3)?
2. What is the nurse's role in supporting Edith from a physical, psychological and social perspective?
3. What do you think the barriers are to broaching a palliative care discussion with Edith, and how can they be overcome?

THE GOLD STANDARDS FRAMEWORK (GSF)

The Gold Standards Framework (GSF) (Thomas et al., 2016), is a systematic, evidence-based approach to optimising care for all patients approaching the end of life. It was originally designed for use in the community by a GP Dr Keri Thomas. It is now used as a way of training practitioners from a range of backgrounds in how to provide a high standard of palliative care.

The GSF (Box 2.3) enables a more in-depth assessment to be made of people with long-term chronic illnesses such as ESPD. The Framework promotes home-based, individualised care, encouraging anticipation of needs. It is a crucial guide to ensure that ESPD is identified promptly and therefore palliative care is initiated early on.

BOX 2.3   THE COPD GOLD STANDARDS FRAMEWORK (GSF) PROGNOSTIC INDICATOR GUIDANCE

- Recurrent hospital admissions (at least three in last 12 months due to ESPD)
- MRC grade 4/5
- Severe disease (e.g. FEV1 <30% predicted), with persistent symptoms despite optimal therapy, too unwell for surgery or pulmonary rehab
- Fulfils long-term oxygen therapy criteria (PaO2<7.3kPa)
- ITU/NIV during hospital admission

Other factors – e.g. right heart failure, anorexia, cachexia, >6 weeks steroids in preceding six months, palliative medication for breathlessness, or still smoking

---

PALLIATIVE CARE

In ESPD the overlap between the acute phase and palliative phase is blurred; the GSF helps healthcare professionals recognise when a person is reaching the palliative phase and thus initiate palliative care. Treatment and interventions for those with ESPD in the palliative stage can cross over with what might be deemed as 'active treatment'; however, the primary aim here is to reduce the impact and severity of the symptoms. In Edith's case, it is clear that she is moving towards the palliative stage. Specific indicators include right-sided heart failure and recurrent hospital admissions, while issues such as an inability to concentrate on everyday tasks, and worsening breathlessness despite optimal treatment, show a general decline that should trigger end of life discussions and planning.

NURSING MANAGEMENT IN THE PALLIATIVE PHASE

One of the most important aspects of ESPD management is smoking cessation. However, it is debatable whether this is appropriate in palliative care; the pleasurable aspects of smoking need to be balanced against the detrimental effect on breathing. Smoking cessation has been shown to have a positive effect on survival rates

(Anthonisen et al., 2005); however, some would argue that it is needless to encourage smoking cessation in end of life (Seamark et al., 2007). In Edith's case, occasional smoking gives her a sense of relief as it brings some normality into her day; however, during severe episodes of breathlessness, smoking becomes too taxing.

Currently, there are no curative treatments available for ESPD, except in rare cases lung transplantation. Pharmacological interventions are often aimed at reducing symptoms and improving overall quality of life for patients with ESPD.

Although not guaranteed to cure, antibiotics (oral, intravenous and nebulised) can be useful to tackle infective exacerbations of ESPD, and thus reduce symptoms such as fatigue and mucus production (Miravitlles and Anzueto, 2017). From the case study, Edith takes long-term prophylactic antibiotics to reduce the risk of frequent chest infections while specific medications are tailored to each branch of chronic pulmonary disease. First line therapy for COPD involves inhaled bronchdilators – for example, salubutamol to reduce airflow limitation (GOLD, 2017; NICE, 2010). Recommendations for restrictive disease such as idiopathic pulmonary fibrosis have less of a conclusive evidence base (NICE, 2017). However, perfenidone (an anti-fibrotic agent) is emerging as an effective treatment to slow the decline in lung function and subjective experience of breathlessness (Noble et al., 2016; NICE, 2013). There are many more pharmacological treatments for chronic lung diseases that are not within the scope of this chapter. However, other interventions mentioned below can be applied to varying end stage pulmonary diseases depending on the specific clinical presentation and symptoms.

Chest physiotherapy can also be used to loosen and suction excessive secretions, particularly common in cystic fibrosis. Other medications that are particularly used in the final stages of the disease include benzodiazepines such as lorazepam, to reduce the anxiety associated with breathlessness. Benzodiazepines are thought to alter the emotional aspect of breathlessness and decrease the respiratory response in respiratory failure (NICE, 2016), while the general anxiolytic effects are often used to reduce the psychological impact of ESPD (Rodriguez-Roisin and Garcia-Aymerich, 2014).

The use of opioids in advanced lung disease is disputed. A systematic review by Jennings et al. (2002) concluded that oral or parenteral opioids had a positive effect on the patient's experience of breathlessness. More recently, a Cochrane review found only low quality evidence in support of this argument, concluding that further research is required (Barnes et al., 2016). However, morphine is still commonly used in current practice for breathlessness, particularly in the last days/hours of life. Usually administered subcutaneously, morphine can settle the person's breathing, which may have become irregular and rapid at times, while having a calming effect.

The majority of acute treatment requires hospitalisation. Even when the patient is in the last year of life, infective exacerbations are usually managed on a medical ward because of the need for IV antibiotics. Once it has been discussed that the patient is EoL, a hospice can provide the appropriate level of care (palliative oxygen therapy, morphine, etc.), or the person can be cared for at home with specialist palliative care nurses and GP monitoring.

OXYGEN THERAPY

While commonly being used during acute hospital admissions, long-term oxygen can be used in chronic hypoxia as the person reaches the palliative stage. Chronic hypoxia affects all organs in the body and is strongly associated with pulmonary hypertension, and in severe cases altered cognition (Kent et al., 2011). Two ground-breaking trials (NOTTG, 1980; MCWP, 1981) provide evidence to show that long-term oxygen therapy (LTOT) extends life expectancy. However, a more recent randomised trial of LTOT found no reduction in mortality in those with moderately low oxygen levels, nor was there any noted benefit to the patient's quality of life (LTOTT, 2016). Despite extremely limited evidence in cystic fibrosis and restrictive lung diseases, the British Thoracic Society (BTS) recommend LTOT in hypoxaemia to prevent associated complications such as pulmonary hypertension, which worsens overall prognosis (Hardinge et al., 2015).

LTOT is usually prescribed for at least 15 hours daily to correct hypoxaemia, while palliative oxygen therapy (POT) is the term used for oxygen administration aimed at relieving the sensation of refractory breathlessness (Hardinge et al., 2015). However, it does not always have the desired effect (Tsara, 2008); a controlled trial examining POT found no symptomatic benefit for the relief of breathlessness and questioned its use in palliative settings, given side effects such as nasal dryness (Abernethy et al., 2010). The BTS therefore advise that oxygen should only be administered when the patient meets the criteria of hypoxaemia. However, they do allow for judgements to be made on an individual basis (Hardinge et al., 2015).

Oxygen therapy in patients with pulmonary disease is sometimes described as a 'comforter' because it has the advantage of reducing anxiety during exacerbations and can enhance social integration by improving mobilisation (Kelly and Maden, 2014; Goldbart et al., 2013). Oxygen administration as a comforter may be associated with other comfort care approaches such as mouth care, therapeutic treatment that maximises a patient's wellbeing. Conversely, it can also be seen as restricting, embarrassing and fear inducing – a sign of severe disease progression (Gruffydd-Jones et al., 2007; Kelly and Maden, 2014). LTOT/POT administration should therefore be a holistic decision. This means that it is based on the individual's preferences and the psychological elements of the therapy are to be accounted for as well as the physical benefits. A nasal cannula is the more common form of oxygen administration in palliative care due to patient comfort and tolerance. Venturi facemasks are used when a controlled concentration of oxygen is needed, or at the patient's request. See Figure 2.3 for the various options of oxygen administration in ESPD. In Edith's case, ambulatory oxygen was used to maintain adequate oxygenation on exertion. However, the cylinder was cumbersome to move, which in some ways negates its benefits.

While oxygen administration is used to counterbalance hypoxia, non-invasive ventilation (NIV) is used to facilitate the exhalation of a greater proportion of carbon dioxide reducing hypercapnia (Rabec et al., 2011). The use of NIV in palliative care is controversial. Carlucci et al. (2012) state that NIV eases breathlessness,

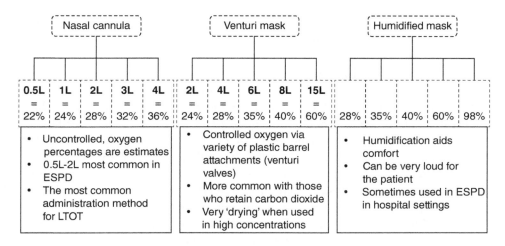

Figure 2.3   Oxygen administration options in ESPD

therefore improving symptomatic experience. Moreover, Nava et al. (2013) found that NIV reduces opioid use in breathlessness, helping maintain good cognition, whereas others argue that NIV protracts the dying process and extends suffering (Curtis et al., 2007). Regardless, some people do not tolerate NIV, or an MDT decision is made not to escalate a person to assisted ventilation. Overall, the amount of acute oxygen intervention is based on the patient's stability, physical health, and most importantly their preferences.

NON-MEDICAL SUPPORTIVE INTERVENTIONS

Non-medical supportive interventions such as chest physiotherapy can be used during acute exacerbations, and are particularly common in end stage cystic fibrosis (Chapman et al., 2005). From another perspective, pulmonary rehabilitation can be used to improve the patient's tolerance of breathlessness with gentle exercise of the limbs. It also educates and empowers patients to self-manage and use the techniques at home (BTS/ACPRC, 2009). Physiotherapists teach breathing techniques such as optimal shoulder positioning for inspiratory effort, or pursed lip breathing to reduce the respiratory rate. Trials have found that intensive pulmonary rehabilitation can reduce in-patient length of stay, lower re-admission rates and improve exercise tolerance in the end stages of the disease (Griffiths et al., 2000; Seymour et al., 2010; Enfield et al., 2010). Qualitative research shows that pulmonary rehabilitation reduces anxiety-related breathlessness and improves the patient's functional independence (de Sousa Pinto et al., 2013; Williams et al., 2009). Patients with ESPD often require further mobility aids as their condition deteriorates; physiotherapists are involved in assessing these needs, especially as part of going home. Occupational therapists recommend adaptations to the living environment to reduce the person's effort in daily activities and promote community management. Wheeled walking devices and perching stools can support the person's independence while easing their symptoms. For Edith, the provision of a downstairs commode is essential as it enables her to live downstairs and therefore remain in the house that has been adapted for her disabled son.

In the palliative phase of ESPD, breathing and relaxation techniques can help ease breathlessness, depression and anxiety (Valenza et al., 2014). Another favourable practice is the use of a hand-held fan to the face. Some hypothesise that stimulation of the trigeminal nerve branches by cool air reduces breathlessness and can be useful in conjunction with other interventions (Booth et al., 2008; Schwartzstein et al., 1987). Some may turn to alternative medicine or complementary therapy; review of acupuncture in pulmonary disease has found that it can reduce breathlessness and improve quality of life (Coyle et al., 2014). Others argue that eucalyptus oil reduces the number of exacerbations (Worth et al., 2009), while menthol may relieve perceived breathlessness due to its anti-tussive (cough relieving), analgesic and bronchodilator properties (Galeotti et al., 2002; Millqvist et al., 2012). Nonetheless, the limited evidence base behind many supportive interventions necessitates that each management plan should be centred on what works for the individual patient. For Edith, being outdoors had a significant effect on reducing her breathlessness; however, this method is dependent on other people, as she needed someone to help her outside.

Help from family and friends can be invaluable to the person with ESPD. They can offer support in a range of ways, from encouragement with smoking cessation in the early days of illness to calming anxiety at the end stage. Often they provide the majority of informal care in the community as the person becomes both physically and psychologically dependent on others.

PSYCHOSOCIAL ASPECTS OF PALLIATIVE CARE

Psychosocial problems due to ESPD play a large part in lowering the person's quality of life. Anxiety and depression are frequently seen in this patient group, but often remain undiagnosed (Pumar et al., 2014).

Anxiety-related breathlessness is a challenging symptom to manage; research has found that physiologically anxiety-related rapid breathing causes shallow breaths which significantly worsen the person's breathlessness (O'Donnell et al., 2007). There is growing evidence that breathlessness is closely linked with the limbic system, which is involved in regulating emotions. However, the overall neurological processes need more detailed mapping; the evidence guiding treatment for breathlessness-related anxiety is inconclusive (Parshall et al., 2012), though cognitive behavioural therapy (CBT) may be helpful (Heslop et al., 2016). Benzodiazepines can be used short term to reduce anxiety, but have been associated with increased mortality in severe pulmonary disease (Ekström et al., 2014).

Long-term, uncontrolled panic and anxiety can lead to more frequent hospital admissions (Dahlén and Janson, 2002). This pattern of anxiety is often complicated by embarrassment and social withdrawal (Bellamy and Booker, 2011). As the disease progresses, physical symptoms combined with the psychological aspects become disabling; people no longer have the strength to go out or enjoy life's pleasures, shrinking their social circle into loneliness (Disler et al., 2014). Edith admitted to experiencing anxiety, and for her, embarrassment is a major barrier to socialising, particularly because of the oxygen cylinder.

Closely linked with social isolation and anxiety in the palliative phase is depression (Hill et al., 2008). The relationship between ESPD, anxiety and depression is convoluted; each individual experience is different. However, risk factors for depression in ESPD include frequent hospital admissions and lack of social support (Hill et al., 2008); symptoms often have a damaging effect on the person's overall functioning (Cully et al., 2006; van Manen et al., 2002). Depression is often attributed to a sense of loss and grief in advanced ESPD, as the person becomes more disabled and increasingly dependent on others. Guilt can also contribute if there is a history of smoking, particularly during episodes of acute breathlessness (Gysels and Higginson, 2011). This has a marked impact on quality of life and is associated with reduced physical activity (Hill et al., 2008). Treatment for depression usually involves anti-depressants (mostly SSRIs); there is less rigorous evidence to support psychological therapies for depression in ESPD; however, patient education has been shown to have some positive effects (Cafarella et al., 2012).

TRANSITION FROM PALLIATIVE TO END OF LIFE CARE

As the illness progresses towards the end stage, the last few weeks can become very difficult for the person and their family to cope with psychologically. The physical symptoms of end stage ESPD often induce hopelessness (Giacomini et al., 2012). Denial is common, and death may be rarely discussed. The progression of ESPD to the end of life can be long; patients often see their illness as a 'way of life', which hinders end of life conversations. This is exacerbated by poor recognition of the palliative stage by healthcare professionals. Patients and professionals can be reluctant to acknowledge the downward trajectory of repeated hospital admissions and worsening symptom severity. The 'unpredictability' of ESPD can cause much stress and worry for caregivers as the patient's condition fluctuates. Healthcare professionals need to involve and support the family through the ups and downs of ESPD and ensure honest conversations prepare those supporting the patient (Ek et al., 2015). Such challenges for relatives can also lead to social problems; for example, Edith's deterioration has led to her husband Michael needing to take more time off work to support her and their disabled son, John.

A review of advance care planning (ACP) in ESPD found the erratic nature of pulmonary disease to act as a barrier to end of life conversations; recovery post exacerbation can mislead those involved that difficult conversations can wait (Patel et al., 2012). Despite Edith's worsening condition, she was noticeably anxious and fearful, reluctant to discuss future events. Detering et al. (2010) highlight how ACP also greatly impacts family members as they have more confidence that the care delivered is derived from the patient's preferences.

The impact of psychological distress related to ESPD can be extremely detrimental to the person's wellbeing. The biopsychosocial aspects of ESPD are inextricably entwined; a truly holistic approach is needed from all healthcare professionals to help guide the person through the palliative stages of the condition.

END OF LIFE CARE PLANNING

Advance care planning is a central part of end of life care, despite the difficulty in engaging with the patient about end of life. The nurse may draw on experience and refined communication skills to assess the patient and family's views on end of life care preferences. Studies show that these conversations rarely take place in practice; barriers range from the patient's lack of readiness to face end of life decisions, to healthcare professional's difficulty in determining the appropriate time to start the conversation (Tavares et al., 2017). Sinclair et al. (2017) suggest nurse-led, facilitated advance care planning significantly improves the occurrence of such conversations.

Part of the nurse's duty of care involves discussing the subject of resuscitation in ESPD; while potentially causing challenges, the team have a responsibility to work in the patient's best interests. 'Do not attempt resuscitation' orders may be implemented in hospital and in the community; however, proper recognition and communication of the palliative stage are crucial to give a sense of choice and empowerment. This allows advance directives, which can be particularly valuable if the person chooses to decline certain treatments and/or states a preferred place of care.

As time went on, Edith agreed to a community DNAR form with her GP as it became clearer than her condition was worsening and would continue to deteriorate.

END OF LIFE CARE

In the care of people with ESPD the fine line between active treatment and palliative/EoL care becomes especially blurred. Decisions are often made on an individual basis, depending on the severity of the patient's symptoms. For Edith, her ambulatory oxygen developed into palliative oxygen and was worn most of the day; she now felt more comfortable with it on as it gave her reassurance that she was still having some 'treatment'. Edith's mobility was increasingly limited due to fatigue and shortness of breath and she began to spend most of her time on her sofa bed asleep. The persistent symptom of breathlessness was managed with palliative treatment, as discussed previously, including small doses of oral morphine liquid. Her husband Michael supported her, with the help of carers in the morning to assist with a gentle wash and to change her pyjamas. This increased sleepiness is a natural part of the dying process.

As the body's normal functions begin to slow down, nutritional requirements lessen. Appetite and thirst decrease and the person often does not want to eat or drink very much. This can be hard for the family and empathetic conversations need to support those close to the dying person. Swallowing difficulties can arise and the person may need to have softer food options and only manage small sips of liquid. In Edith's case, she could only manage sips of fortified milkshake through a straw. She had also begun wearing an incontinence pad, as she no longer had control over her bladder and bowel. As the days went on, these functions lessened and her urine output was minimal. Hygiene needs remain essential in end of life care, but great care is needed to ensure the least possible distress to the person.

During this time, there is often withdrawal from social interactions and reduced engagement with those near them, moving towards prolonged drowsiness. In ESPD, this stage of dying varies greatly. The gradual loss of consciousness may occur over a number of days, or can happen within the space of minutes to hours. Breathing changes ensue, such as shallow breathing, and eventually long pauses between breaths. If severe breathlessness continues, morphine and or midazolam can be used to reduce distress, most commonly as a continuous subcutaneous infusion via a syringe driver. Excessive secretions are common, which cannot be coughed up and lead to 'rattling' breathing. This can be particularly distressing for relatives, as they may fear the person is drowning. Medication to reduce the secretions (e.g. glycopyrronium bromide) can be given alongside any other medications needed in the syringe driver or as bolus doses.

The person can also be laid on their side to prevent the secretions from gathering in the back of the throat; however, excellent mouth care is most important. If possible, the family can be involved in providing essential care such as mouth care and assisting with washing, which may also bring them some comfort as well as the patient. Supportive interventions such as these play a vital role in caring for someone with ESPD; the nurse must be very patient and listen to what is truly important to the person and their family. Above all, it is fundamental that compassion underpins nursing care for those with ESPD.

In her final days, Edith was cared for at home, supported by district nurses, the specialist palliative care team, community respiratory nurses, her GP, and of course, her family. The team of healthcare professionals had discussed an advance care plan with Edith and her family in her last few weeks, which enabled Edith to die at home as she preferred. However, this is not always the case in ESPD. Some patients continue to receive active and invasive treatment up until death without sufficient palliative support or the chance to discuss their preferences for end of life care.

CONCLUSION

This chapter has provided a detailed view of the complexity of ESPD and its origins as a disease commonly referred to as COPD. Tracing the pathophysiology of lung disease, the chapter has demonstrated how nurses can detect changes in the patient's condition indicating deterioration and the onset of ESPD. The chapter has also looked at the nursing management of patients with ESPD during its transition from acute intervention, the palliative phase and end of life care. One of the complex and challenging features of ESPD for palliative care practitioners is lack of distinction between acute intervention, palliative care and end of life. The chapter has demonstrated how the fine line between active treatment and palliative/EoL care becomes blurred. Decisions about whether a person has reached the palliative stage are often made on an individual basis, depending on the severity of the patient's symptoms.

It has been shown that the patient's illness trajectory from becoming palliative to end stage can be protracted with the patient perceiving their illness as a 'way of life'. This can hinder end of life conversations and advance care planning. In these circumstances, wherever possible, practitioners need to consider the transition from palliative to end of life as soon as the answer to the surprise question is, 'No, I would not be surprised if the patient died in three months' time.' However, in many patients with ESPD, the end of life can come very quickly if they fail to recover sufficiently from an acute infective illness. Some of the issues related to ESPD, such as breathlessness, are described and discussed in the next chapter, which focuses on patients with end stage heart failure (ESHF). The reader will find some of the text in Chapter 3 similar to but different to the issues discussed in this chapter.

A version of this chapter was published in the *International Journal of palliative Nursing*, Volume 23, Issue 10, 486–95. Under the title 'Palliative care for people living with end-stage pulmonary disease' with kind permission of SAGE Publications, Ltd.

ANSWERS TO REFLECTIVE EXERCISE 2.1

1. Recurrent hospital admissions, MRC grade 5, smoking, heart failure, palliative medication for breathlessness and cachexia.
2. The nurse's role includes managing Edith's breathlessness with breathing techniques and medication, monitoring symptoms for exacerbations, referring to other services (e.g. dieticians), liaising with Edith's consultant/GP to improve medication management (e.g. monitoring inhaler effectiveness), and giving Edith the time and space to express how she feels about her situation.
3. Barriers to palliative care discussions may include Edith's determination to stay strong to look after her son, reluctance to accept her deterioration, anxieties about death, the healthcare professional's eagerness to focus on trying to solve Edith's problems rather than looking at the whole picture. These could be overcome by including Edith's whole family in discussions about the future, having frank discussions with Edith and allowing her to express her true worries about the end of life, and having a discussion as a team of healthcare professionals to acknowledge Edith's deterioration and make sure everyone is on the same page.

REFERENCES

Aaron, S.D., Stephenson, A.L., Cameron, D.W. and Whitmore, G.A. (2015) 'A statistical model to predict one-year risk of death in patients with cystic fibrosis.' *Journal of Clinical Epidemiology, 68* (11): 1336–45.

Abdo, W.F. and Heunks, L.M.A. (2012) 'Oxygen-induced hypercapnia in COPD: myths and facts.' *Critical Care, 16* (5): 323.

Abernethy, A.P., McDonald, C.F., Frith, P.A., Clark, K., et al. (2010) 'Effect of palliative oxygen versus room air in relief of breathlessness in patients with refractory dyspnoea: a double-blind, randomised controlled trial.' *The Lancet, 376* (9743): 784–93.

Anthonisen, N.R., Skeans, M.A., Wise, R.A., Manfreda, J., Kanner, R.E. and Connett, J.E. (2005) 'The effects of a smoking cessation intervention on 14.5- year mortality: a randomized clinical trial.' *Annals of Internal Medicine, 142* (4): 233–9.

Arshad, S.H. and Babu, K.S. (2008) *Asthma – The Facts*. Oxford: Oxford University Press.

Barnes, H., McDonald, J., Smallwood, N. and Manser, R. (2016) 'Opioids for the palliation of refractory breathlessness in adults with advanced disease and terminal illness.' *Cochrane Database of Systematic Reviews 3*: CD011008.

Bellamy, D. and Booker, R. (2011) *Chronic Obstructive Pulmonary Disease in Primary Care*. 4th ed. London: Class Publishing.

Booth, S., Moosavi, S.H. and Higginson, I.J. (2008) 'The etiology and management of intractable breathlessness in patients with advanced cancer: a systematic review of pharmacological therapy.' *Nature Clinical Practice Oncology, 5* (2): 90–100.

British Lung Foundation (BLF) (2016) *The Battle for Breath: The Impact of Lung Disease in the UK*. Available at https://cdn.shopify.com/s/files/1/0221/4446/files/The_Battle_for_Breath_report_48b7e0ee-dc5b-43a0-a25c-2593bf9516f4pdf?70457014513584722 54&_ga=2.50418464.823874507.1519144891-1700414640.1519144891, accessed 20 February 2018.

British Lung Foundation (BLF) (2017) *Idiopathic Pulmonary Fibrosis Statistics*. Available at www.blf.org.uk/support-for-you/idiopathic-pulmonary-fibrosis-ipf/statistics, accessed 15 February 2017.

British Thoracic Society/Association of Chartered Physiotherapists in Respiratory Care (BTS/ACPRC) (2009) *Concise BTS/ACPRC Guidelines: Physiotherapy Management of the Adult, Medical, Spontaneously Breathing Patient*. British Thoracic Society Reports, Vol. 1, No. 1. London: British Thoracic Society.

Cafarella, P. A., Effing, T. W., Usmani, Z. and Frith, P. A. (2012) 'Treatments for anxiety and depression in patients with chronic obstructive pulmonary disease: A literature review.' *Respirology, 17*(4): 627–38.

Carlucci, A., Guerrieri, A. and Nava, S. (2012) 'Palliative care in ESPD patients: is it only an end-of-life issue?' *European Respiratory Review, 21*: 347–54.

Chapman, E., Landy, A., Lyon, A., Haworth, C. and Bilton, D. (2005) 'End of life care for adult cystic fibrosis patients: facilitating a good enough death.' *Journal of Cystic Fibrosis, 4* (4): 249–57.

Coyle, M., Shergis, J., Tzu-Ya Huang, E., Guo, X., et al. (2014) 'Acupuncture therapies for chronic obstructive pulmonary disease: a systematic review of randomized, controlled trials.' *Alternative Therapies in Health and Medicine, 20* (6): 10–23.

Cully, J.A., Graham, D.P., Stanley, M.A., Ferguson, C.J., et al. (2006) 'Quality of life in patients with chronic obstructive pulmonary disease and comorbid anxiety or depression.' *Psychosomatics, 47* (4): 312–19.

Currie, G.P. and Chetty, M. (2011) 'Diagnosis', in G.P. Currie (ed.), *ABC of COPD*. 2nd ed. Chichester: John Wiley & Sons.

Curtis, J.R., Cook, D.J., Sinuff, T., White, D.B., et al. (2007) 'Noninvasive positive pressure ventilation in critical and palliative care setting: understanding the goals of therapy.' *Critical Care Medicine, 35* (3): 932–9.

Dahlén, I. and Janson, C. (2002) 'Anxiety and depression are related to the outcome of emergency treatment in patients with obstructive pulmonary disease.' *Chest, 122* (5): 1633–7.

Detering, K.M., Hancock, A.D., Reade, M.C. and Silvester, W. (2010) 'The impact of advance care planning on end of life care in elderly patients: randomised controlled trial.' *British Medical Journal, 340*: c1345.

Disler, R.T., Green, A., Luckett, T., Newton, P.J., et al. (2014) 'Experience of advanced chronic obstructive pulmonary disease: metasynthesis of qualitative research.' *Journal of Pain and Symptoms Management, 48*, >6,: 1182–99.

Effros, R. M. and Swenson, E. R. (2016) 'Acid-Base Balance', in V. C. Broaddus, R. J. Mason, J. D. Ernst, T. E. King, Jr., S. C. Lazarus, J. F. Murray, J. A. Nadel, J. S. Slutsky and M. B. Gotway (eds) *Murray & Nadel's Textbook of Respiratory Medicine* E-Book. 6th ed. Philadelphia: Elsevier Saunders.

Ek, K., Andershed, B., Sahlberg-Blom, E. and Ternestedt, B. (2015) '"The unpredictable death" – the last year of life for patients with advanced COPD: relatives' stories.' *Palliative and Supportive Care, 13* (5): 1213–22.

Ekström, M.P., Bornefalk-Hermansson, A., Abernethy, A.P. and Currow, D.C. (2014) 'Safety of benzodiazepines and opioids in very severe respiratory disease: national prospective study.' *British Medical Journal, 348*: g445.

Enfield, K., Gammon, S., Flyod, J., Falt, C., et al. (2010) 'Six-minute walk distance in patients with severe end-stage COPD: association with survival after inpatient pulmonary rehabilitation.' *Journal of Cardiopulmonary Rehabilitation and Prevention, 30* (3): 195–202.

Galeotti, N., Di Cesare Mannelli, L., Mazzanti, G., Bartolini, A. and Ghelardini, C. (2002) 'Menthol: a natural analgesic compound.' *Neuroscience Letters, 322* (3): 145–8.

Gardiner, C., Gott, M., Payne, S., Small, N., et al. (2010) 'Exploring the care needs of patients with advanced COPD: an overview of the literature.' *Respiratory Medicine, 104* (2): 159–65.

Giacomini, M., DeJean, D., Simeonov, D. and Smith, A. (2012) 'Experiences of living and dying with COPD: a systematic review and synthesis of the qualitative empirical literature.' *Ontario Health Technology Assess Series, 12* (13): 1–47.

Global Initiative for Chronic Obstructive Lung Disease (GOLD) (2017) *Global Strategy for the Diagnosis, Management and Prevention of Chronic Obstructive Pulmonary Disease,* 2017 Report. Available at http://goldESPD.org/gold-2017-global-strategy-diagnosis-management-prevention-ESPD, accessed 21 December 2016.

Gnanapandithan, K. and Agarwal, R. (2012) 'Respiratory failure', in S.K. Jindal (ed.) *Handbook of Pulmonary and Critical Care Medicine.* New Delhi: Jaypee Brothers, Medical Publishers.

Goldbart, J., Yohannes, A.M., Woolrych, R. and Caton, S. (2013) '"It is not going to change his life but it has picked him up": a qualitative study of perspectives on long term oxygen therapy for people with chronic obstructive pulmonary disease.' *Health and Quality of Life Outcomes, 11*: 124–32.

Griffiths, T.L., Burr, M.L., Campbell, I.A., Lewis-Jenkins, V., Mullins, J., Shiels, K., Turner-Lawlor, P.J., Payne, N., Newcombe, R.G., Ionescu, A.A., Thomas, J. and Tunbridge, J. (2000) 'Results at 1 year of outpatient multidisciplinary pulmonary rehabilitation: a randomised controlled trial.' *Lancet, 355*(9201): 362–8.

Gruffydd-Jones, K., Langley-Johnson, C., Dyer, C., Badlan, K. and Ward, S. (2007) 'What are the needs of patients following discharge from hospital after an acute exacerbation of chronic obstructive pulmonary disease (ESPD)?' *Primary Care Respiratory Journal, 16* (6): 363–8.

Gysels, M.H. and Higginson, I.J. (2011) 'The lived experience of breathlessness and its implications for care: a qualitative comparison in cancer, ESPD, heart failure and MND.' *BMC Palliative Care, 10* (15).

Hardinge, M., Annandale, J., Bourne, S., Cooper, B., et al. (2015) 'BTS guidelines for home oxygen use in adults.' *Thorax*, 70: i1–i43.

Health and Safety Executive (HSE) (2017) Asbestos-related diseases [online]. Available at www.hse.gov.uk/statistics/causdis/asbestosis/asbestos-related-disease.pdf, accessed 23 June 2018.

Heslop, K., Stenton, C., Newton, J., Carrick-Sen, D., et al. (2016) 'A randomised controlled trial of cognitive behavioural therapy (CBT) delivered by respiratory nurses to reduce anxiety in chronic obstructive pulmonary disease (ESPD).' *European Respiratory Journal*, 68 (suppl. 60): OA289.

Hill, K., Geist, R., Goldstein, R.S. and Lacasse, Y. (2008) 'Anxiety and depression in end-stage ESPD.' *European Respiratory Journal*, 31 (3): 667–77.

Jennings, A.L., Davies, A.N., Higgins, J.P.T., Gibbs, J.S.R. and Broadley, K.E. (2002) 'A systematic review of the use of opioids in the management of dyspnoea.' *Thorax*, 57: 939–44.

Kelly, C.A. and Maden, M. (2014) 'How do respiratory patients perceive oxygen therapy? A critical interpretative synthesis of the literature.' *Chronic Respiratory Disease*, 11 (4): 209–28.

Kent, B.D., Mitchell, P.D. and McNicholas, W.T. (2011) 'Hypoxemia in patients with ESPD: cause, effects, and disease progression.' *International Journal of Chronic Obstructive Pulmonary Disease*, 6: 199–208.

Leivseth, L., Nilsen, T.I.L., Mai, X., Johnsen, R. and Lanbghammer, A. (2012) 'Lung function and anxiety in association with dyspnoea: the HUNT study.' *Respiratory Medicine*, 106 (8): 1148–57.

The Long-Term Oxygen Treatment Trial Research Group (LTOTT) (2016) 'A randomized trial of long-term oxygen for COPD with moderate desaturation.' *New England Journal of Medicine*, 375 (17): 1617–27.

Medical Council Working Party (MCWP) (1981) 'Long term domiciliary oxygen therapy in chronic hypoxic cor pulmonale complicating chronic bronchitis and emphysema. Report of the Medical Research Council Working Party.' *Lancet*, 1 (8222): 681–6.

Millqvist, E. Ternesten-Hasséus, E. and Bende, M. (2012) 'Inhalation of menthol reduces capsaicin cough sensitivity and influences inspiratory flows in chronic cough.' *Respiratory Medicine*, 107 (3): 433–8.

Miravitlles, M. and Anzueto, A. (2017) 'Chronic respiratory infection in patients with chronic obstructive pulmonary disease: what is the role of antibiotics?' *International Journal of Molecular Sciences*, 18 (7): 1344.

Mitchell, D., Wells, A., Spiro, S. and Moller, D. (eds) (2012) *Sarcoidosis*. Boca Raton, FL: Taylor and Francis.

Nakamura, Y. and Suda, T. (2015) 'Idiopathic pulmonary fibrosis: diagnosis and clinical manifestations.' *Clinical Medicine Insights: Circulatory, Respiratory and Pulmonary Medicine*, 9 (suppl 1): 163–71.

Nathan, S.D., du Bois, R.M., Albera, C., Bradford, W.Z., et al. (2015) 'Validation of test performance characteristics and minimal clinically important difference of the 6-minute walk test in patients with idiopathic pulmonary fibrosis.' *Respiratory Medicine*, 109 (7): 914–22.

National Institute for Clinical Excellence (NICE) (2010) *Chronic Obstructive Pulmonary Disease in over 16s: Diagnosis and Management*. Clinical guideline [CG101]. Manchester: NICE.

National Institute for Clinical Excellence (NICE) (2013) *Pirfenidone for Treating Idiopathic Pulmonary Fibrosis*. Available at www.nice.org.uk/guidance/ta282/chapter/1-guidance, accessed 10 September 2017.

National Institute of Clinical Excellence (NICE) (2016) *Clinical Knowledge Summaries: Palliative Care – Dyspnoea* [online]. Available at: https://cks.nice.org.uk/palliative-care-dyspnoea#!scenariorecommendation:5> , accessed: 9 July 2017.

National Institute for Clinical Excellence (NICE) (2017) *Idiopathic Pulmonary Fibrosis in Adults: Diagnosis and Management.* Available at www.nice.org.uk/guidance/CG163/chapter/1-Recommendations#prognosis, accessed 9 September 2017.

Nava, S., Ferrer, M., Esquinas, A., Scala, R., et al. (2013) 'Palliative use of non-invasive ventilation in end-of-life patients with solid tumours: a randomised feasibility trial.' *The Lancet Oncology, 14* (3): 219–27.

Noble, P.W., Albera, C., Bradford, W.Z., Costabel, U., et al. (2016) 'Pirfenidone for idiopathic pulmonary fibrosis: analysis of pooled data from three multinational phase 3 trials.' *European Respiratory Journal, 47*(1): 243–53.

Nocturnal Oxygen Therapy Trial Group (NOTTG) (1980) 'Continuous or nocturnal oxygen therapy in hypoxemic chronic obstructive lung disease: a clinical trial.' *Annals of Internal Medicine, 93* (3): 391–8.

O'Donnell, D., Banzett, R., Carrieri-Kohlman, V., Casaburi, R., et al. (2007) 'Pathophysiology of dyspnea in chronic obstructive pulmonary disease: a roundtable.' *Proceedings of the American Thoracic Society, 4* (2): 145–68.

Parshall, M.B., Schwartzstein, R.M., Adams, L., Banzett, R.B., et al. (2012) 'An official American Thoracic Society statement: update on the mechanisms, assessment, and management of dyspnea.' *American Journal of Respiratory and Critical Care Medicine, 185* (4): 435–52.

Patel, K., Janssen, D.J.A. and Randell Curtis, J.A. (2012) 'Advance care planning in COPD.' *Respirology, 17* (1): 72–8.

Pumar, M.I., Gray, C.R., Walsh, J.R., Yang, I.A., Rolls, T.A. and Ward, D.L. (2014) 'Anxiety and depression – important psychological comorbidities of COPD.' *Journal of Thoracic Disease, 6* (11): 1615–31.

Rabec, C., Rodenstein, D., Leger, P., Rouault, S., Perrin, C. and Gonzalez-Bermejo, J. (2011) 'Ventilator modes and settings during non-invasive ventilation: effects on respiratory events and implications for their identification.' *Thorax, 66* (2): 17–18.

Rennard, S.I. and Vestbo, J. (2006) 'ESPD: The dangerous underestimate of 15%.' *The Lancet, 367* (9518): 1216–19.

Rodriguez-Roisin, R. and Garcia-Aymerich, J. (2014) 'Should we exercise caution with benzodiazepine use in patients with COPD?' *European Respiratory Journal, 44* (2): 284–6.

Schwartzstein, R.M., Lahive, K., Pope, A., Weinberger, S.E. and Weiss, J.W. (1987) 'Cold facial stimulation reduces breathlessness induced in normal subjects.' *The American Review of Respiratory Disease, 136* (1): 58–61.

Seamark, D.A, Seamark, C.J. and Halpin, D.M.G. (2007) 'Palliative care in chronic obstructive pulmonary disease: a review for clinicians.' *Journal of the Royal Society of Medicine, 100* (5): 225–33.

Seymour, J.M., Moore, L., Jolley, C.J., Ward, K., et al. (2010) 'Outpatient pulmonary rehabilitation following acute exacerbations of ESPD.' *Thorax, 65* (5): 423–8.

Sinclair, C., Auret, K.A., Evans, S.F., Williamson, F., et al. (2017) 'Advance care planning uptake among patients with severe lung disease: a randomised patient preference trial of a nurse-led, facilitated advance care planning intervention.' *BMJ Open, 7* (2). doi: 10.1136/bmjopen-2016–013415.

Snell, N., Strachan, D., Hubbard, R., Gibson, J., et al. (2016) 'Burden of lung disease in the UK: findings from the British Lung Foundation's "respiratory health of the nation" project.' *European Respiratory Journal, 48* (suppl. 60): PA4913.

de Sousa Pinto, J.M., Martín-Nogueras, A.M., Morano, M.T., Macêdo, T.E., Arenillas, J.I. and Troosters, T. (2013) 'Chronic obstructive pulmonary disease patients' experience with pulmonary rehabilitation: a systematic review of qualitative research.' *Chronic Respiratory Disease, 10* (3):141–57.

Stenton, C. (2008) 'The MRC breathlessness scale.' *Occupational Medicine, 58* (3): 226–7.

Tavares, N., Jarrett, N., Hunt, K. and Wilkinson, T. (2017) 'Palliative and end-of-life care conversations in COPD: a systematic literature review.' *European Respiratory Journal Open Research*, *3* (2): 00068–2016.

Thomas, K., Armstrong Wilson, J. et al. (2016) *The Gold Standards Framework Proactive Identification Guidance (PIG)*. 6th ed. Shrewsbury: National Gold Standards Framework Centre in End of Life Care.

Tsara, V., Serasli, E., Katsarou, Z., Tsorova, A., Christaki, P. (2008) 'Quality of life and social-economic characteristics of Greek male patients on long term oxygen therapy.' *Respiratory Care*, *53* (8): 1048–53.

Valenza, M.C., Valenza-Peña, G., Torres-Sánchez, I., González-Jiménez, E., Conde-Valero, A. and Valenza-Demet, G. (2014) 'Effectiveness of controlled breathing techniques on anxiety and depression in hospitalized patients with ESPD: a randomized clinical trial.' *Respiratory Care*, *59* (2): 209–15.

van Manen, J.G., Bindels, P.J., Dekker, F.W., IJzermans, C.J., van der Zee, J.S., Schadé, E. (2002) 'Risk of depression in patients with chronic obstructive pulmonary disease and its determinants.' *Thorax*, *57* (5): 412–16.

Vestbo, J. (2010) 'Clinical assessment of ESPD', in N.A. Hanania and A. Sharafkhaneh (eds), *ESPD: A Guide to Diagnosis and Clinical Management*. New York: Humana Press.

Williams, V., Bruton, A., Ellis-Hill, C. and McPherson, K. (2009) 'The effect of pulmonary rehabilitation on perceptions of breathlessness and activity in ESPD patients: a qualitative study.' *Primary Care Respiratory Journal*, *19*: 45–51.

Worth, H., Schacher, C. and Dethlefsen, U. (2009) 'Concomitant therapy with Cineole (Eucalyptole) reduces exacerbations in COPD: a placebo-controlled double-blind trial.' *Respiratory Research*, *10* (1): 69.

FURTHER READING

British Lung Foundation (BLF) (2018) *Support for You*. Available at www.blf.org.uk/support-for-you, accessed 3 March 2018.

Higginson, I.J., Reilly, C.C. Bajwah, S., Maddocks, M., Costantini, M. and Gao, W. (2017) 'Which patients with advanced respiratory disease die in hospital? A 14-year population-based study of trends and associated factors.' *BMC Medicine*, 15: 19.

Pinnock, H., Kendall, M., Murray, S.A., Worth, A., et al. (2011) 'Living and dying with severe chronic obstructive pulmonary disease: multi-perspective longitudinal qualitative study.' *British Medical Journal*, 342: d142.

3

PALLIATIVE CARE FOR PEOPLE WITH END STAGE HEART FAILURE (ESHF)

SHARON GRIMSDALE

LEARNING OUTCOMES

- Describe the pathophysiology of end stage heart failure (ESHF)
- Describe and discuss diagnosis, treatment and symptom management
- Provide an account of supportive interventions for patients with ESHF

INTRODUCTION

The purpose of this chapter is to describe in detail the changes that take place in the heart as we age and the effects caused by disease, as well as treatment. The chapter will discuss diagnosis, symptom control and clinical management issues. Moreover, the chapter will look at the situation whereby, as a result of disease and often many years of malfunction, the person's heart failure becomes advanced or end stage and palliative care is required. The chapter will discuss therapeutic interventions that can be taken to improve quality of life using case study material. The case study highlights end of life issues and the changes to symptom management and medication administration required to provide quality palliative care. The types of interventions which are appropriate for people with heart failure are often dependent on the setting in which care takes place, although for many with end stage heart failure palliative measures can be provided in a number of hospital and community contexts. One of the core features of the chapter is the need to understand the symptoms and the pathophysiology causing them in order to initiate a high standard of clinical management. In order to develop a fuller picture of the disease it is necessary to include the experiences of a patient's family members with end of life care.

UNDERSTANDING HEART FAILURE

Cardiovascular disease (CVD) causes more than 150,000 (26%) of all deaths in the UK each year; it is estimated that 42,000 people under the age of 75 in the UK die from CVD each year (ONS, 2017). However, mortality figures for people with long-term illnesses such as heart failure show a decline in the number of people dying due to people living longer long term illnesses such as heart disease, creating a greater need for palliative care when the disease reaches the end stages (Sin et al., 2018). Heart failure is a progressive condition with no cure and high mortality rates (Department of Health, 2016). As we age, the left ventricle of the heart enlarges slightly compared to the amount of work it does, and to an extent a very mild form of heart failure, in the absence of disease, may be considered acceptable. Cardiovascular disease (CVD) is an umbrella term used to describe a range of heart conditions including those arising from hereditary factors and those now common in developing countries such as coronary heart disease, atrial fibrillation, heart failure and stroke. The term heart failure (HF) is often used in relation to other terms to describe the functioning or otherwise of the heart, such as cardiac disease, coronary thrombosis or coronary heart disease. Heart failure relates to the dysfunction of the heart muscle and its internal parts and can occur at any age (BHF, 2002). Considering the work conducted by the heart it is perhaps not unusual to find that as we grow older its efficiency in most people is impaired. Over 400,000 people in England have been diagnosed with heart failure but there are many more undiagnosed cases.

The most common cause of heart failure in the UK is coronary heart disease (NICE, 2003; NHS, 2000; Atienza et al., 2004). This is caused by damage to the heart muscle, usually as a result of a heart attack (BHF, 2002). However, approximately one-third of cases in the UK are a result of hypertensive disease (NHS, 2000). Other precipitating factors include cardiomyopathy, congenital heart disease, valvular disease, obesity, thyroid disease, arrhythmia, some cancer treatments, viral infections and alcohol or recreational drug toxicity (NICE, 2003; BHF, 2002). Overall, HF is defined (SIGN, 1999) as the heart's inability to deliver enough oxygen in the blood to meet the demands required by the metabolising tissues despite normal or increased cardiac filling pressures, therefore reducing the heart's inability to pump effectively (NHS, 2000).

DIAGNOSIS, TREATMENT AND SYMPTOM MANAGEMENT

There are a number of different types of heart failure:

- Left ventricular systolic dysfunction (LVSD)
- Right ventricular systolic dysfunction

- Left or right diastolic dysfunction
- Congestive heart failure
- Heart failure with preserved ejection fraction (HFpEF)

Of these, the most common type is left ventricular systolic dysfunction (LVSD) as this affects the left ventricle, which is the heart's main pumping chamber. This is also known as left ventricular failure (LVF), heart failure with reduced ejection fraction (HFrEF) or heart failure with mid-range ejection fraction (HFmrEF) (Ponikowski et al., 2016).

CLINICAL DIAGNOSIS

Clinical assessment of the patient is paramount to aid diagnosis. The symptoms of heart failure are similar to other conditions and should not be ignored:

- Breathlessness, orthopnoea, paroxysmal nocturnal dyspnoea
- Cough with or without productive phlegm
- Oedema (peripheral, pulmonary, ascites)
- Fatigue, lethargy
- Dizziness
- Weight loss, weight gain, poor appetite
- Constipation
- Confusion
- Dehydration
- Pain (assessment of type of pain, duration and treatment responses)

Assessment should look for the cause of breathlessness such as pulmonary oedema from decompensated heart failure with fluid overload, chest infection, pleural effusion (which could be due to fluid overload or infection, pulmonary embolism or underlying bronchogenic cancer), pulmonary embolism or neoplasm. Many patients with heart failure also have co-existent COPD or asthma as a contributory cause of their breathlessness (Johnson, 2007).

There are two main pathways for heart failure in the UK, acute and chronic. Once heart failure is suspected, a 12-lead ECG should be undertaken. This is to look for arrhythmia, hypertrophy, strain or left bundle branch block. Following the chronic pathway, a negative brain naturetic peptide (BNP) blood test could exclude heart failure diagnosis, although borderline results could not exclude diagnosis (Balion et al., 2006); if the result is positive the patient should be referred for an echocardiogram. This is the gold standard diagnostic tool. It is important to bear in mind those patients with ischaemic heart disease who may have had a cardiac MRI or coronary angiogram which can also identify LVSD. The ejection fraction (EF) can be calculated and patients are classed as mild, moderate or severe. A severe ejection fraction is <35% (NICE, 2010) although new European Society of Cardiology (ESC) guidance (Ponikowski et al., 2016) states that EF<40% is considered significant. This is known as heart failure with reduced ejection fraction (HFrEF).

The most common symptom is shortness of breath, either with exercise or at rest (BHF, 2002; NICE, 2003). Other occurring symptoms include weight gain, peripheral and ascites oedema, lethargy, dizziness, increased nocturnal micturition, nausea, malnourishment and confusion, all with varying severity from day to day (BHF, 2002; NICE, 2003; SIGN, 1999; Stewart and Blue, 2001). The symptoms are identified in four groups according to the New York Heart Association Classification of heart failure (New York Heart Association, 2002). Although the severity of symptoms can be grouped in the NYHA, assessment of prognosis can be difficult as these patients have a high risk of sudden death (NHS, 2000). Patients are assessed according to the NYHA scale but can move from each class on assessment depending on symptoms. The NYHA is used internationally and is helpful for comparing and recording functional status as well as response to therapy. However, it does have limited consistency with an inability to quantify some of the symptoms of HF (National Heart Foundation of New Zealand, 2001; Raphael et al., 2007).

According to the NYHA Classification System (see Box 3.1), it is not uncommon to find that patients with established heart failure who develop chest infections causing breathing to deteriorate to be classified as class II stable heart failure. Depending on the severity of the chest infection and the deterioration of their condition, they could be classified as class III. Alternatively, if a class III patient had a change to medication that improved their symptoms they could move back to class II. Therefore, it may be seen that the NYHA classification table is a useful way of identifying the severity of the patients' symptoms as well as a guide for assessing people with established heart failure. Patients with progressive end stage heart failure would move from class III to class IV as their symptoms and condition progress.

BOX 3.1 WHAT IS THE NYHA CLASSIFICATION SYSTEM?

- It is used to classify symptoms of heart disease
- Systems are graded on how much they limit your functional capacity ranging from Class I (no limitation on activity) to Class IV (symptoms persisting even at rest) with patients unable to undertake any physical activity without discomfort)
- Annual mortality rates increase with each level
- With the system patients can move from one class to another depending on how well or poorly they respond to treatment

For more information on the NYHA Classification system visit: http://www.heart.org/en/health-topics/heart-failure/what-is-heart-failure/classes-of-heart-failure

EXTENDED CASE STUDY 3.1   PETER

Peter, 64 years old, had a history of ischaemic heart disease, having had a myocardial infarction (MI) some 15 years previously. Although there was no family history of heart disease, the MI occurred within hours after a serious stressful event. Peter initially attended a cardiac reha-bilitation programme and life continued until he started to notice his breathing was gradually deteriorating. He started waking during the night, gasping for breath and having to sit on the edge of the bed. He was already using three pillows, and having four pillows made only a slight difference. Peter started to get out of breath having a shower and had to rest to get his breath before getting dried and again before getting dressed. Walking had become limited and Peter noticed more frequent stops to get his breath. He lived in a bungalow so did not have to negoti-ate stairs. He noticed his legs started to swell with mild pitting oedema to the knees. Peter saw his GP and a brain naturetic peptide (BNP) blood test was requested. A positive result of 1560 meant he was referred for a two-week echocardiogram as per NICE guidance (2010). Due to a previous MI he was referred directly for an echocardiogram without the need for BNP testing (NICE, 2014). The echocardiogram showed severe LVSD with an ejection fraction of 30 per cent and some diastolic dysfunction, which prompted a referral to the community heart failure nurse specialist service. Patient access to a heart failure nurse specialist (HFNS) is variable across the country but they can reduce NHS costs, hospital admissions, improve the quality of life and facilitate better communication across primary, secondary and community care (Department of Health, 2016; McKay and Stewart, 2004; Stewart et al., 2002).

On initial assessment in the specialist clinic Peter was assessed as NYHA class III (see Table 3.1). His breathing was stable at rest but impaired on exertion. He had nocturnal breathlessness and was unable to lie flat. He slept in an upright position but had disturbed sleep due to coughing with productive clear phlegm. On chest auscultation he had basal crepitations to left base. Peter was already optimised on ramipril (10mg daily), carvedilol (25mg twice daily) and eplerenone (50mg daily). NICE guidance recommends triple therapy of an angiotensin converting enzyme (ACE) inhibitor (usually ending in 'pril' such as ramipril, enalapril), beta blocker (usually ending in 'lol' – only three are licensed for heart failure, bisoprolol, carvedilol and nebivolol), and an aldosterone antagonist (spironolactone or eplerenone) (NICE, 2014).

Peter was also taking a loop diuretic (furosemide), 80mg in the morning and 40mg in the afternoon. Baseline renal function showed some moderate chronic kidney disease (CKD). He had started to develop exertional chest pain requiring the use of glycerin trinitrate spray (GTN). His pulse was irregular as expected with known atrial fibrillation at a tachycardic rate of 96bpm. Peter was hypotensive with a sitting BP 100/60, standing 106/64. He had some dizziness on standing too quickly. Based on this assessment there was scope to increase his loop diuretic to potentially improve his symptoms by reducing his fluid overload from his chest and peripheral leg oedema and improving the NYHA score back to II. By offloading the excess fluid Peter's blood pressure should also improve and pulse rate should decrease as cardiac output improves. Over the next three months Peter was educated around symptom recognition and medication optimisation. Lifestyle and dietary advice was discussed. Furosemide was increased to 120mg in the morning and 80mg at lunchtime. His breathing had stabilised and mobility had improved. His chest auscultation resolved; peripheral pitting oedema to mid-calf was now mild and Peter was able to sleep on two pillows with no nocturnal breathlessness. He continued to have some exertional breathlessness but was able to walk further than on his initial referral. His chest pain was managed with oral nitrate and his dizziness had settled with an increase in his BP 118/66 sitting, 122/66 standing. Renal function initially deteriorated but later stabilised. Peter felt better in himself and was subsequently discharged back to his GP with an open self-referral should his symptoms deteriorate and an NYHA score of II. He was invited to attend a heart failure exercise programme run at the hospital following British Cardiovascular Society (2017) guidelines but he declined.

Table 3.1   Drugs commonly used in the treatment of heart failure

Loop diuretics	Recommended to improve symptoms and exercise capacity in patients with signs and symptoms of congestion	20–240 mg daily	Further reading
Furosemide		0.5–5 mg daily	
Bumetanide		5–20 mg daily	
Torasemide			
Thiazides		2.5–10 mg daily	
Metolazone		25–100 mg daily	
Hydrochlorothiazide		2.5–10 mg daily	
Bendroflumethazide			
Potassium Sparing		2.5–20 mg daily	
Amiloride			
ACE-I	For symptomatic patients with HFrEF to reduce the risk of HF hospitalisation and death. Used in addition to a Beta blocker	2.5–10 mg daily	AIRE study / HOPE study
Ramipril		2.5–20 mg BD	CONSENSUS / SOLVD
Enalapril		2.5–35 mg daily	
Lisinopril			
ARB	Recommended to reduce the risk of HF hospitalisation and cardiovascular death in symptomatic patients unable to tolerate an ACE-I	4–32 mg daily	CHARM trial
Candesartan		40–160 mg BD	
Valsartan		50–150 mg daily	
Losartan			
Beta blockers	Recommended for patients with stable, symptomatic HFrEF to reduce the risk of HF hospitalisation and death. Used in addition to ACE-I	1.25–10 mg daily	CIBIS II
Bisoprolol		3.125–25 mg BD	MERIT-HF trial
Carvedilol		1.25–10 mg daily	
Nebivolol		12.5–200 mg daily	
Metoprolol succinate (CR/XL)			
MRAs	Recommended for HFrEF who remain symptomatic despite treatment with an ACE-I and beta blocker, to reduce the risk of HF hospitalisation and death	25–200 mg daily	RALES trial
Spironolactone		25–50 mg daily	EMPHASIS-HF/ EPHESUS
Eplerenone			

(Continued)

Table 3.1   (Continued)

If-channel blocker Ivabradine	To reduce the risk of HF hospitalisation or cardiovascular death in symptomatic patients with LVEF 35% in sinus rhythm and a resting heart rate >70bpm despite treatment with an evidence-based beta blocker, who are unable to tolerate or have contra-indications to a beta blocker	5–7.5mg BD	SHIFT trial
ARNI Sacubitril/Valsartan	Recommended as a replacement for an ACE-I to further reduce the risk of HF hospitalisation and death in ambulatory patients with HFrEF who remain symptomatic despite optimal treatment	49/51–97/103 mg BD	PARADIGM-HF trial
Digoxin	Considered in symptomatic patients in sinus rhythm despite treatment with an ACE-I (or ARB), beta blocker and an MRA to reduce the risk of hospitalisation (both all cause and HF hospitalisations)	62.5–250 mcg daily	Digitalis Investigation Group

SUPPORTIVE INTERVENTIONS FOR PATIENTS WITH END STAGE DISEASE

There is evidence to suggest that 30 to 40 per cent of patients with a diagnosis of heart failure will die within a year; thereafter, mortality is less than 10 per cent per year (NICE, 2010; Stewart et al., 2001). Peter had been invited to a heart failure support group which was a local joint working project (Better Together). This project recognised the need to refer patients to palliative care services earlier in their disease progression to achieve the best quality of life (Nordgren and Sorensen, 2003; Maciver and Ross, 2018). Heart failure nurse specialists (HFNS) are experienced practitioners who are familiar with the use of the surprise question, 'Would you be surprised if the patient died in the next 12 months?'. If the nurses were to answer yes to the surprise question then this can help in planning for end of life for patients with heart failure. HFNS are experienced in discussing patients' concerns as well as providing and co-ordinating end of life care (Johnson et al., 2012). The difficulties surrounding the DNA/CPR decision may be the outcome of several weeks' sensitive discussion with patients and families who have not realised they have advanced disease and have unrealistic expectations of CPR. Such discussions require the HFNS to develop advanced communication skills (Department of Health, 2016).

Peter contacted the heart failure nurse specialist service with deteriorating symptoms. He noticed that his breathing had deteriorated at night. He required extra pillows at night, though they had little effect, and he had to sit on the edge of the bed to ease his breathlessness. Breathlessness in patients with heart failure is the most common symptom in the last six months of life, amongst others such as oedema, incontinence, pain and anxiety (Nordgren and Sorensen, 2003). His leg oedema was moderate due to pitting up to the knees. On clinical assessment he had basal crepitations to both bases with a productive cough. Phlegm was white and frothy, ruling out a chest infection. Peter had some left-sided ischaemic chest pain on moderate exertion which was relieved with GTN spray. He developed some palpitations and manual pulse was recorded at 150bpm irregular – he was known to have atrial fibrillation (AF). Peter had no dizziness and no postural hypotension on sitting and standing BP. Weight had increased by 10kg to 90kg since he was last seen by the service.

Following the treatment algorhythm (Ponikowski et al., 2016, see Figure 3.1) Peter was optimised on ramipril, carvedilol and eplerenone (triple therapy). Baseline electrolytes were taken to monitor renal function and potassium levels. Raised potassium can cause abnormal heart rhythms and be an indicator for worsening renal failure, and needed to access best medication treatment. Potassium levels came back at 5.3 (upper end of normal limits) and urea (16.6) and creatinine (154) was stable for Peter and within his usual limits. In view of his symptoms furosemide was increased to 120mg twice daily. An ECG was requested due to raised heart rate levels due to increased cardiac workload but also he had palpitations with irregular rhythm, probably due to AF but it could also indicate an underlying abnormal ventricular rhythm. As part of ESC guidance (Ponikowski et al., 2016) an ECG should be carried out to assess for left bundle branch block (LBBB). Peter's ECG showed AF as expected but he was found to have an LBBB with a QRS of 145msec. Blood pressure remained around 100 systolic.

As his weight was over 85kg, increasing carvedilol to 50mg BD could have been considered but it was not possible to do so in view of hypotension. Ivabradine is used to control heart rate but is of no benefit in AF. Digoxin is used for end stage heart failure and is useful to control heart rate in the context of AF and has been shown to reduce hospitalisation but has no benefit on mortality or morbidity outcomes (Digitalis Investigation Group, 1997).

On further review, following an increase in furosemide, Peter's symptoms showed no improvement. He was struggling to settle in bed and when reclining at rest he felt he was suffocating. Positions that might help were discussed, such as sitting upright, and leaning forward over a table as this opens the lung capacity from the back. There is some evidence that a cool fan blowing towards the face can help the individual feel less suffocated. A study of the use of oxygen showed it was of no prognostic benefit although further research was recommended (Clark et al., 2015).

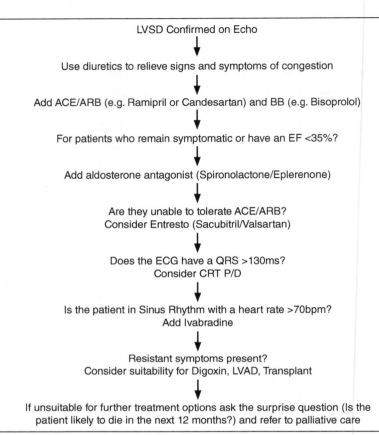

Figure 3.1   Treatment Algorhythm

Source: Adapted from Ponikowski et al. 2016

Despite increased diuretics Peter started struggling with urinary incontinence. He could not stand quickly without becoming unsteady and light headed, and mobility was restricted due to worsening oedema. Repeat renal function tests showed slightly worsening urea and creatinine blood levels as expected. Peter felt his condition was deteriorating and chest auscultation revealed crackles to left mid-zone that was persistent to right base. His potassium was now 3.5mmols. Peter was already optimised on maximal furosemide therapy orally as well as on eplerenone (potassium sparing) and could have been swapped to spironolactone to give larger doses. However, he had initially tried it but was intolerant due to gynacomastia. Amiloride (potassium sparing diuretic) was commenced at 2.5mg OD in addition to his current treatment. Peter found the incontinence a struggle and embarrassing. He was sleeping in an armchair propped up with pillows and his legs on a stool no higher than his waist. He felt most comfortable in this position. He became more lethargic as his heart was struggling with the fluid overload, reduced cardiac output and fast heart rate. Peter was also struggling to complete sentences without having to stop to get his breath. Peter had been on amiloride for two days but noticed his legs had started leaking. The fluid in his thighs was starting to seep through the skin and his weight had increased to 98kg. Peter rang an on-call out-of-hours GP and was admitted to hospital over the weekend. It was decided that Peter would not be resuscitated if he had a cardiac arrest. He was commenced on IV furosemide and catheterised for urinary incontinence and to monitor fluid output. Diuretics are mainly used to remove fluid retention, providing rapid symptomatic relief (Cowie and Zaphirou, 2002). They are not known to reduce mortality and doses are altered depending on patient symptoms such as breathing, renal function and fluid retention.

Fluid intake was restricted to 1.5 litres per day. After three days of furosemide IV, Peter had lost 6kg. He was placed back on oral diuretics and discharged with follow-up by the HFNS. A cardiologist appointment was brought forward due to hospital admission for heart failure, LBBB and suitability for cardiac resynchronisation therapy – CRT-P (pacemaker) or CRT-D (defibrillator).

Peter was not keen on hospital admission. He was asked for his thoughts on his symptoms and he recognised he was not getting any better. When compared to how he was 12 months previously there was a marked deterioration. He felt unable to leave the house. Walking from one room to the next was such an effort and he felt exhausted afterwards. He was sleeping more and nodding off while watching his favourite television programmes. Over the next month Peter became more withdrawn. Initially he had been a happy, smiley man who liked to joke. He had taken an interest in his heart failure and became a patient voice for the British Heart Foundation. Seeing Peter now was heartbreaking. He confided that he did not wish to be a burden on his family. His wife had become his full-time carer and had taken to sleeping on the sofa in case he woke during the night and needed assistance. He was unable to wash himself without help. After washing, Peter would fall asleep for three hours. He had to have a strip wash as he was unable to get his heavy oedematous legs over the bath. If he had got in the bath and sat down he would not have been able to get back up. Peter's abdomen had become more distended with ascites. He was having his leg dressings changed by the district nurses on a daily basis, due to his odema, unlike some medical conditions, compression bandaging is contraindicated in heart failure. He had a pressure relieving cushion to sit on and he was encouraged to stand and gently move around frequently to relieve and change pressure. Peter was losing interest in food and his appetite was decreasing. He felt full all the time. His fluid weight was increasing and not his dry body weight. You could see his shoulders were becoming thinner but his abdomen was getting larger. Peter was referred to a dietitian for supplements to build his calorie intake.

When first diagnosed, a healthy diet had been recommended but now, to boost calorie intake, dietary changes such as full cream milk and eating little and often were advised. Medication initially given to improve and support heart function such as ACE inhibitors were stopped to allow the prescribing of additional diuretics in order to alleviate fluid overload (Cowie and Zaphirou 2002). Metolazone 2.5mg OD was initiated (off licence) for three days. His weight was 102kg and he remained adamant that he did not want to go into hospital, despite being told that his heart failure was deteriorating. Recognising that patients are nearing the end of their lives is very challenging and requires sensitive communication and a lot of clinical skill to initiate the introduction of palliative care (Taylor et al., 2018). Specialist nurses such as HFNS are experienced at initiating discussion about end of life care and advanced care planning, which often includes discussion of resuscitation (Johnson et al., 2012; Stewart and Blue, 2001; Blue et al., 2001; Ackroyd, 2005). However, Peter made the decision he no longer wanted to be resuscitated. He was open and honest and did not want to die at home. He had previously attended a heart failure support group at the local hospice and had liked the surroundings. He said he did not want his wife to remember him in his chair in the front room when he died and think of his death every time she looked at the chair. Peter was happy to receive hospice care and this became his preferred place of care and the place he wished to spend the rest of his life.

As Peter's symptoms deteriorated during the last year of life, an integrated team with cardiology, palliative care and the general practitioner were able to help prevent unwanted hospital admissions at the end of life (Johnson et al., 2012). Peter's weight was increasing despite increasing diuretic therapy. His renal function was deteriorating. It is common for peaks and troughs to occur in heart failure trajectory, which can often make death appear sudden. The Gold Standards Framework on end of life care suggests frequent hospital admissions in the last year are suggestive of deterioration. However, the role of HFNS is hospital avoidance and medication management.

At this stage in Peter's condition (Taylor et al., 2018) it was recognised that in view of the prognosis Peter was not suitable for a CRT device or assessment for a heart transplant or a left ventricular assist device (LVAD). He was becoming increasingly breathless even at rest. He remained chesty with basal crepitations despite the addition of metolazone. His odematous legs had developed cellulitis due to leaking and continued being dressed daily by the district nurses. They were very painful and Peter struggled to stand. The amount of bandaging required to absorb the fluid made walking unsteady. The oedema made his feet feel numb. Referral to palliative care for pain management was discussed, to which he agreed. Pain is common in end of life for heart failure patients and is not just due to oedema in the legs but also in the abdomen due to ascites and excess fluid causing severe discomfort when carrying out simple tasks like bending down or sitting forward. This pushes up the lungs, increasing breathlessness. Other causes of pain include peripheral circulatory pain and neuropathic pain due to the oedema pressing on the nerves (Johnson, 2007). Despite Peter's ischaemic background, he had no chest pain as this was controlled with nitrates. However, he started to suffer with muscularskeletal chest tenderness due to over-inflation of the lungs trying to ease breathlessness. At times he was hyperventilating and becoming anxious when he could not breathe. A small dose of oromorph was suggested to assist with his breathing and would also be useful in assessing his pain threshold (Health Education England, 2016). Sublingual lorazepam is often used for paroxysmal nocturnal dyspnoea. It is usually taken sublingually so that if any side effects develop or breathlessness eases the lorazepam can be removed easily and the patient feels more in control.

Peter was struggling to sleep at night. He was frightened to go to sleep in case he didn't wake up. This caused more anxiety. He found getting in and out of bed increasingly difficult and very uncomfortable. He started sleeping in the chair with his feet elevated on a buffet stool. His restricted position and reduced movement had started to cause pressure area breakdown on his sacrum. His weight continued to increase to 113kg and oedema increased to scrotal and waist with some moderate pitting to lower abdomen and lower back. He had also developed some mild pitting oedema to his forearms. Admission to the hospice for subcutaneous furosemide (BHF, 2015; Grimsdale, 2014) was discussed with Peter. This could have been done in the community but his preferred place of care was adhered to. His renal function had deteriorated further with his urea being 28 and creatinine 250. Clinical signs showed he was dying. His nitrate medication and statin levels were discontinued as they were now considered of no prognostic benefit. Beta blockers continued to maintain heart rate control of his AF. His ramipril had been stopped previously due to deteriorating renal function and to maintain blood pressure. Peter was placed on a syringe driver with furosemide.

As Peter was in the hospice he was started on morphine tablets for pain control with oromorph for breakthrough pain and breathlessness as per local guidelines (Health Education England, 2016). Peter developed a uraemic itch consistent with end stage renal function and diuretic therapy. He became more lethargic. He started to become increasingly agitated, not just from the uraemic itch but because he was unable to get comfortable and because of anxiety related to breathlessness and cerebral irritation. Discussions with his wife and family took place as they found it hard to see Peter agitated and uncomfortable. They found it distressing to see Peter confused. He had deteriorated rapidly and symptoms clinically suggested the last days of life. It was agreed that patient comfort would take priority. No further blood tests were necessary, weight did not require monitoring and only essential medications were given to maintain comfort. Peter required regular opiates and in the interests of his quality of life it was agreed that morphine be administered via a syringe driver with an antiemetic drug and emetic medication. Peter's family were present throughout and Peter finally settled. Syringe drivers are often sited in the abdomen. However, this restricts absorption with oedematous patients. Alternative sites include upper chest, shoulders or upper arms (Grimsdale, 2014). The use of syringe drivers helps to control symptoms and prevent episodes of breakthrough pain, providing consistent analgesic control, especially at the end of life when patients may become unable to take oral medication. Peter became more drowsy and took sips of fluids only. He became unable to tolerate oral medications and relied on furosemide and morphine via a syringe driver for symptom management. Mouth care, hygiene and pressure area care are very important with all patients approaching end of life. Diuretics can cause dry mouth, and family members can assist with mouth care if they wish to be involved. Peter died peacefully with his family present in his preferred place of care.

Other things to consider in providing end of life care for people with heart failure include:

- Deactivation of internal cardiac defibrillator (ICD or CRT-D) (Beattie, 2013)
- Advance care planning
- Preferred place of care
- Preferred place of death

- Do not attempt resuscitation
- Anticipatory medications (for symptomatic management with specialist input and support)
- Access to benefits (personal independence payment, attendance allowance)
- Access to palliative care team
- Access to multidisciplinary team such as occupational therapy, social services, aids and adaptations
- Lasting power of attorney
- Organ and tissue donation
- Advance decision making

Mental Capacity Act 2005 (Bradford, Airedale, Wharfedale and Craven Palliative Care Managed Clinical Network, 2015)

CONCLUSION

Patients with ESHF when they reach the end of life experience symptoms similar to other patients with non cancer conditions, such as pain, anxiety, fatigue and agitation. Peter's family were grateful for the amount of support they received from all the professional staff who provided their expertise including the heart failure nurse but also from the hospice staff. Peter's family appreciated that he lived longer than they had initially expected and that there had been so many episodes when they felt he would die but were relieved that he managed to pull round and become stable. Peter's death, there have been numerous changes made in the way people with ESHF are treated. Delete died further interventions treating. Insert new sentence The treatment of high risk patients with severe LVSD like Peter delete NYHA CLASSES II-IV. After end of life care insert has improved by the introduction of drugs such as Enestro (McMurray et al 2014) full stop. Insert new sentence drugs like this delete to, ... reduce mortality and improve the quality of the patients life. Delete and investigating the link between heart failure and iron deficiency (ponikoski et al 2016) continue to develop. Heart failure is a long-term condition which continues to have a poor prognosis and early access to palliation should be paramount. Some heart failure patients with LVSD have access to HFNS but all heart failure patients should have access to palliative care services in the last year of life. Although Peter died in the hospice, access to hospice at home, Marie Curie nurses and specialist palliative care teams would all have been made available if his choice had been to stay at home. The BHF funded a successful two-year pilot on the delivery of intravenous (IV) diuretics in the community (Beattie, 2013) that could now have been considered for Peter. The trajectory of heart failure remains unpredicatable and referral to palliative care is often inconsistent and remains poor (Department of Health, 2016; Voon et al., 2017). Without the involvement of HFNS, the average time from palliative care referral to death is around 21 days (Bakitas et al., 2013). *Our Commitment to You for End of Life Care* (Department of Health, 2016) addressed some of the key issues and commitments to ensure care improvement for all, including heart failure, which has been recognised not just in the UK but in other parts of the world such as Japan (Kurozumi et al., 2018).

REFERENCES

Ackroyd, R.A. (2005) 'Medically futile resuscitation: can it ever be justified?' *European Journal of Palliative Care, 12* (5): 207–9.

Atienza, F., Anguita, M., Martinez-Alzamora, N., Osca, J., et al. (2004) 'Multicenter randomised trial of a comprehensive hospital discharge and outpatient heart failure management program.' *The European Journal of Heart Failure*, 6: 643–52.

Bakitas, M. et al. (2013) 'Palliative care consultations for heart failure patients: how many, when and why?' *Journal of Cardiac Failure*, 19 (3): 193–201.

Balion, C., Santaguida, P., Hill, S., Worster, A., et al. (2006) 'Testing for BNP and NT-proBNP in the diagnosis and prognosis of heart failure.' *Evidence Report/Technology Assessment*, 142: 1–7.

Beattie, J. (2013) *ICD Deactivation at the End of Life: Principles and Practice. A Discussion Document for Healthcare Professionals*. Birmingham: British Heart Foundation.

Blue, L., Lang, E., McMurray, J.J.V., Davie, A.P., et al. (2001) 'Randomised controlled trial of specialist nurse intervention in heart failure.' *British Medical Journal*, 323 (7315): 715–18.

Bradford, Airedale, Wharfedale and Craven Palliative Care Managed Clinical Network (2015) *Advance Care Plan Personal Preferences and Wishes for Future Care*. Version 1, February.

British Cardiovascular Society (2017) *The BACPR Standards and Core Components for Cardiovascular Disease Prevention and Rehabilitation 2017*. 3rd ed. London: BACPR.

British Heart Foundation (BHF) (2002) *Living with Heart Failure*. London: British Heart Foundation.

British Heart Foundation (BHF) (2015) *Treating Heart Failure Patients in the Community with Intravenous Diuretics*. London: British Heart Foundation.

Clark, A.L., Johnson, M., Fairhurst, C., Torgerson, D., et al. (2015) 'Does home oxygen therapy (HOT) in addition to standard care reduce disease severity and improve symptoms in people with chronic heart failure? A randomised trial of home oxygen therapy for patients with chronic heart failure.' *Health Technology Assessment*, 19 (75): 1–120.

Cowie, M.R. and Zaphirou, A. (2002) 'Management of chronic heart failure.' *British Medical Journal*, 325 (7361): 422–5.

Department of Health (2016) *Our Commitment to You for End of Life Care: The Government Response to the Review of Choice in End of Life Care*. Available at www.gov.uk/government/uploads/system/uploads/attachment_data/file/536326/choice-response.pdf, accessed 31 May 2018.

Digitalis Investigation Group (1997) 'The effect of digoxin on mortality and morbidity in patients with heart failure.' *New England Journal of Medicine*, 336: 525–33.

Gold Standards Framework (2018) *Advance Care Planning*. Available at www.goldstandardsframework.org.uk/advance-care-planning, accessed 31 JulyMay 2018.

Grimsdale, S. (2014) *Guideline for Administration of Subcutaneous Furosemide in the Community Setting in Bradford and Airedale*. Available at www.palliativecare.bradford.nhs.uk/Documents/SC%20Furosemide%20Policy.pdf, accessed 31 May 2018.

Health Education England (2016) *A Guide to Symptom Management in Palliative Care. Version 6*. Yorkshire and Humber Palliative End of Life Care Groups supported by Health Education England.

Johnson, M. (2007) 'Management of end stage cardiac failure.' *Postgraduate Medical Journal*, 83: 395–401.

Johnson, M., Nunn, A., Hawkes, T., Stockdale, S. and Daley, A. (2012) 'Planning for end-of-life care in heart failure: experience of two integrated cardiology-palliative care teams.' *British Journal of Cardiology*, 19: 71–5.

Kurozumi, Y., Oishi, S., Sugano, Y., Sakashita, A., et al. (2018) 'Design of a nationwide survey on palliative care for end stage heart failure in Japan.' *Journal of Cardiology*, 71 (2): 202–11.

Maciver, J. and Ross, H. (2018) 'A palliative approach for heart failure end-of-life care.' *Current Opinion in Cardiology*, 33 (2): 202–7.

McKay, I. and Stewart, S. (2004) 'Optimising the day to day management of patients with chronic heart failure', in S. Stewart and L. Blue (eds), *Improving Outcomes in Chronic Heart Failure: Specialist Nurse Intervention from Research to Practice*. 2nd ed. London: BMJ Books.

McMurray, J.J.V., Packer, M., Desai, A.S., Gong, J., et al. (2014) 'Angiotensin-neprilysin inhibitors versus enalapril in heart failure.' *The New England Journal of Medicine*, 371 (11): 993–1004.

National Heart Foundation of New Zealand (2001) 'A guideline for the management of heart failure: health professionals guide.' *New Zealand Medicine Journal*, 110: 99–107.

New York Heart Association (2002) *New York Heart Association Classification System: The Stages of Heart Failure*. Heart Failure Society of America.

NHS (2000) 'Heart failure' in *National Service Framework for Coronary Heart Disease*. London: Department of Health.

NICE (2003a) *Management of Heart Failure*. London: National Institute for Clinical Excellence.

NICE (2003b) *Chronic Heart Failure – Management of Chronic Heart Failure in Primary and Secondary Care*. Guideline 5. London: National Institute for Clinical Excellence.

NICE (2010) *Chronic Heart Failure in Adults: Management*. London: National Insititute for Clinical Excellence.

NICE (2014) *Acute heart failure: diagnosis and management*. Available at: www.nice.org.uk/guidance/cg187/chapter/1-Recommendations#initial-pharmacological-treatment, accessed October 2018.

Nordgren, L. and Sorensen, S. (2003) 'Symptoms experienced in the last six months of life in patients with end-stage heart failure.' *European Journal of Cardiovascular Nursing*, 2: 213–17.

Office of National Statistics (2017) *Deaths from diseases of the cardiovascular system and ischaemic heart disease 2010–2016*. Availble at: www.ons.gov.uk/peoplepopulationandcommunity/birthsdeathsandmarriages/deaths/adhocs/007824deathsfromdiseasesofthe-cardiovascularsystemandischaemicheartdisease2010to2016, accessed October 2018.

Ponikowski, P., Voors, A.A., Anker, S.D., Bueno, H. et al. (2016) '2016 ESC guidelines for the diagnosis and treatment of acute and chronic heart failure: the Task Force for the diagnosis and treatment of acute and chronic heart failure of the European Sociaty of Cardiology (ESC).' *European Heart Journal*, 37 (27): 2129–200.

Raphael, C., Briscoe, C., Davies, J., Whinnett, Z., et al. (2007) 'Limitations of the New York Heart Association functional classification system and self-reported walking distances in chronic heart failure.' *Heart*, 93: 476–82.

SIGN (1999, modified 2002) *Diagnosis and Treatment of Heart Failure Due to Left Ventricular Systolic Dysfunction*. Edinburgh: Scottish Intercollegiate Guidelines Network.

Sin, J., Henderson, C., Spain, D., Cornelius, V. et al. (2018). 'Health interventions for family carers of people with long term illness: A promising approach?' *Clinical Psychology Review*, 60: 09–125.

Stewart, S. (2004) 'Increased health care utilisation and costs: heart failure in the 21st century', in S. Stewart and L. Blue (eds) *Improving Outcomes in Chronic Heart Failure: Specialist Nurse Intervention from Research to Practice*. 2nd ed. London: BMJ Books.

Stewart, S. and Blue, L. (2001) *Improving Outcomes in Chronic Heart Failure: Specialist Nurse Intervention from Research to Practice*. 2nd ed. London: BMJ Books.

Stewart, S., Jenkins, A., Buchan, S., McGuire, A., Capewell, S. and McMurray, J. (2002) 'The current cost of heart failure to the National Health Service in the UK.' *European Journal of Heart Failure*, 4: 361–71.

Stewart, S., MacIntyre, K., Hole, D., Capewell, S. and McMurray, J. (2001) 'More "malignant" than cancer? Five-year survival following a first admission for heart failure.' *European Journal of Heart Failure*, 3: 315–22.

Taylor, P., Crouch, S., Howell, D., Dowding, D. and Johnson, M. (2018) 'Change in physiological variables in the last two weeks of life: an observational study of hospitalised adults with heart failure.' *Journal of Pain and Symptom Management*, 55 (5): 1335–40.

Voon, V., Chew, S., Craig, C., White, D., et al. (2017) 'Can we do better in improving end of life care and symptom control in end stage heart failure?' *Heart* (Suppl 6), 103: A1–A39.

FURTHER READING

Acute Infarction Ramipril Efficacy (AIRE) Study Investigators (1993) 'Effect of ramipril on mortality and morbidity of survival of acute myocardial infarction with clinical evidence of heart failure.' *The Lancet*, 342: 821–8.

CONSENSUS Trial Study Group (1987) 'Effects of enalapril on mortality in severe congestive heart failure: results of the co-operative North Scandinavian Study (Consensus).' *New England Journal of Medicine*, 326 (23): 1429–35.

Heart Outcomes Prevention Evaluation (HOPE) Study Investigators (2000) 'Effects of an angiotensin-converting enzyme inhibitor, ramipril, on cardiovascular events in high risk patients.' *New England Journal of Medicine*, 342: 145–53.

Hjalmarson, A., Goldstein, S., Fagerberg, B., Wedel, H., et al. (1999) 'Effect of metoprolol CR/XL in chronic heart failure: metolprolol CR/XL randomised intervention trial in congestive heart failure (MERIT-HF).' *The Lancet*, 353 (9169): 2001–7.

Lechat, P., Hulot, J., Escolano, S., Mallet, A., et al. (2001) 'Heart rate and cardiac rhythm relationships with bisoprolol benefit in chronic heart failure in CIBIS II trial.' *Circulation*, 103: 1428–33.

McMurray, J., Ostergren, J., Swedberg, K., Granger, C., et al. (2003) 'Effects of candesartan in patients with chronic heart failure and reduced left ventricular systolic function taking angiotensin-converting-inhibitors: the CHARM-ADDED trial.' *The Lancet*, 362 (9386): 767–71.

Packer, M., Bristow, M., Cohn, J., Colucci, W., et al. (1996) 'The effect of carvedilol on morbidity and mortality in patients with chronic heart failure.' *New England Journal of Medicine*, 334: 1349–55.

Pitt, B., Zannad, F., Remme, W.J., Cody, R., Castaigne, A., Perez, A. (1999). 'The effects of Spironolac-tone on morbidity and mortality in patients with severe heart failure. Randomised Aldactone Evaluation Study (RALES)'. *New England Journal of Medicine*, 341 (10): 709–17.

SOLVD Investigators (1991) 'Effect of enalapril on survival in patients with reduced left ventricular ejection fractions and congestive heart failure.' *New England Journal of Medicine*, 325: 293–302.

Swedberg, K., Komajda, M., Bohm, M., Borer, J., et al. (2010) 'Ivabradine and outcomes in chronic heart failure (SHIFT): a randomised placebo-controlled study.' *The Lancet*, 376 (9744): 875–85.

Zannad, F., McMurray, J., Krum, H., van Veldhuisen, et al. (2011) 'Eplerenone in patients with systolic heart failure and mild symptoms.' *New England Journal of Medicine*, 364 (1): 11–21.

4

PALLIATIVE CARE FOR PEOPLE WITH MULTIPLE SCLEROSIS

JOHN COSTELLO

LEARNING OUTCOMES

- Identify the common symptoms and different subtypes of multiple sclerosis (MS)
- Describe the experiences patients often encounter in living with the disease and its unique nature
- Consider the palliative care as it relates specifically to MS
- Describe the role of the nurse in supporting patients and families at the end of life

---

INTRODUCTION

The purpose of this chapter is to provide information on the pathophysiology of MS and some of the common symptoms and subtypes of the disease. It also looks at the various treatments used to control relapses and prevent symptoms such as muscle spasm through the use of prescribed medication, massage and the use of medicinal cannabis (sativex). Moreover, consideration is given to the unique nature of MS and how each individual with the disease has their own experiences. It does this through the use of case studies which examine the problematic nature of diagnosis and the importance of quality of life and living with the disease. The case studies are used as an anchor within the chapter to help focus the rest of the symptom management and patient experiences. Due to the complex nature of MS, patients may be referred to a neuro-rehabilitation team or Multiple Sclerosis specialist practice nurse for symptom management. As the disease progresses, social care can be provided to assist with Activities of Daily Living (ADL).When the disease reaches the palliative phase, social care support often continues in conjunction with palliative services.

As the case study will illustrate, palliative care is focused on providing optimal care, not just for the patient but the family caregivers who are provided with various amounts of support from professional caregivers and organisations such as the MS Society and MS Trust. Finally, the chapter looks at palliative care end of life, highlighting a number of challenges for healthcare professionals.

BACKGROUND

Multiple sclerosis (MS) is a serious degenerative neurological condition that involves damage to the body's neurological system, specifically the myelin sheath covering the nerve (Alonso et al., 2007). The global prevalence of MS is increasing with an estimated 2.3 million people diagnosed in 2013, representing an increase of 0.2 million since 2008. In the UK it has been estimated that over 100,000 people are living with MS (Alonso et al., 2007). These figures are likely to underestimate the growing problem which is confounded by the high incidence of misdiagnosis, which is a very challenging and persistent problem that has significant consequences for patients and healthcare professionals (Solomon and Corboy, 2017). The condition often begins between the ages of 20 and 50 and is more common in women than men on a ratio of three females to every one male (3:1) (MS Society, 2017). The damage to the nerve cell involves a breakdown in the outer covering of the nerve, known as demyelination. Demyelination is the key pathophysiology of the disease, which can lead to numerous physical and psychological problems that impact on ADL, resulting from the neurological damage.

SYMPTOM RECOGNITION AND EFFECTS

MS is a long-term illness characterised by periods of remission and relapses of symptoms often referred to as attacks. These episodes can cause pain, lack of mobility, incoordination and a number of psychological issues such as anger and depression. One of the features of these relapses is their lack of predictability. Practitioners working with people with MS need to be aware not only of the disease progression but also the impact it has on the individual patient. In the palliative phase of the illness, the relapses may become more frequent, severe and debilitating. One of the consistent features of MS throughout the disease progression is fatigue, which is more than feeling tired and involves a range of psychological issues like frustration and anxiety which can be treated and the person supported.

BOX 4.1   MAIN SYMPTOMS OF MS

- Fatigue
- Muscle spasticity, weakness and ataxia (balance problems)
- Visual disturbances
- Speech difficulties (dysarthria)
- Swallowing problems (dysphagia)
- Cognitive impairment
- Depression
- Anxiety and frustration
- Unstable mood
- Pain, sensation (hypoesthesia, and tingling – paraesthesia)
- Bowel problems (incontinence, diarrhoea and constipation)
- Urinary frequency and/or retention

Box 4.1 provides an overview of the main symptoms associated with MS. MS leads to difficulties in coordination, problems with balance and mobility, eyesight, musculoskeletal problems, bladder difficulties, speech problems and tingling sensations in the peripheral limbs. There are also a wide range of other problems, sometimes referred to as invisible, that are associated with MS that become part of the more physical symptoms. These include fatigue, which is ever present throughout the condition and can be severe during attacks. Many people with MS report that they experience a combination of symptoms at the same time.

Some of the symptoms illustrated in Box 4.1, such as speech difficulties, may occur in the initial stages of MS as a result of dysarthria and thereafter not become troublesome to the patient as they adapt to the difficulty in mobilising the tongue in the mouth. Similarly, visual problems can be accommodated and, although initially worrying, can be less of a problem than symptoms such as muscle spasticitiy which can cause pain, discomfort and lack of mobility. Muscle spasticity can be a consistent feature and one that the chapter will discuss in more detail due to the problem in managing this distressing symptom. Other symptoms such as hypoestesia and paraesthesia and bowel disturbances can result from the use of certain medications such as buscapan, used to control muscle spasm. The psychological effects of MS, such as anxiety, mood changes and cognitive impairment, affect some people more than others. Much depends on the individual's attitude, personality and level of tolerance. Moreover, the support provided by others and the care and attention they receive can make a significant difference to individual wellbeing. In Greater Manchester the MS Centre exists as an information provider and source of social support for people with MS. As a day facility it provides people with MS and their caregivers with a place where they can receive treatment and social support, very important in the management of symptoms. One of the universal issues about symptom management in MS is its variability. People with MS may not experience the range and severity of some symptoms like visual disturbances. Most would agree that muscle spasticity is a prevalent feature and one that causes pain and anxiety. It can also become a distressing problem giving rise to other symptoms such as anxiety and severe frustration. Due to the unpredictable nature of MS, not everyone experiences all these symptoms and certainly not at one time.

DIFFERENT FORMS OF MS

MS takes several forms and has different subtypes with new symptoms either occurring in isolated attacks (relapsing forms) or building up over time (progressive forms) – see Box 4.2. A recurrence of the symptoms once they have remained dormant for several months or years is referred to as an attack. Between attacks, symptoms may disappear completely; however, permanent neurological problems often remain, especially as the disease advances. Despite the underlying cause being ambiguous, the pathology of the disease is focused on dysfunction of the immune system or failure of the myelin-producing cells. Proposed causes for this include genetics and environmental factors, with viral infection being a likely trigger. Another likely trigger is stress, which like other illnesses such as stroke can precede the onset of symptoms (Methley et al., 2014). MS is usually diagnosed based on the presenting signs and symptoms and the results of supporting medical tests.

BOX 4.2 SUBTYPES OF MS

1. Progressive-relapsing MS: Characterised by steady decline from onset with superimposed attacks
2. Secondary progressive MS: Characterised by initial relapsing-remitting MS that suddenly begins to decline without periods of remission
3. Primary progressive MS: Characterised by a steady increase in disability without attacks
4. Relapsing-remitting MS: Characterised by unpredictable attacks which may or may not have permanent decline followed by periods of remission (Methley et al., 2014).

DIAGNOSING MS

MS is commonly diagnosed between the ages of 20 and 40, although it can be diagnosed in children and in later life. A confirmed diagnosis, which matches the symptoms to MS, happens after the patient has had two isolated episodes or attacks. In terms of Dennis and his experiences, it is necessary to say that despite the signs of MS no two people have exactly the same symptoms (Solomon and Corboy, 2017).

CASE STUDY 4.1   DENNIS

Dennis was a 27-year-old who lived at home with his parents. His father (Eric) was diagnosed with MS in his 20s, around the same age Dennis began to have symptoms of MS. It seemed to start very innocently. He was aware that MS had a tendency to be familial and he had looked up what the symptoms were online. He put it out of his head, arguing with himself that it was not worth worrying about since he could not do anything about it anyway. He had an older brother who did not have MS, married with a baby girl. Dennis enjoyed his job working for a university as an IT technician and was very competent at his job. He had an active social life and was passionate about football, playing for a local Sunday league team. He enjoyed the games and the social life that existed in the pub after the matches.

It was just after his 28th birthday that he recalled feeling lethargic, but he put this down to the amount of drinking at his birthday party and the subsequent hangover. He started to experience blurred vision, although at first it was hard to say exactly what he was experiencing except that he did not feel as though he was seeing things properly. He also started to feel frustrated at work, becoming unable to sort out problems which he normally would have dealt with well. Perhaps most noticeably, he seemed to lose his football skills and suddenly felt as though he had two left feet. He thought he was just going through a low period and carried on as normal.

In the next few weeks, things started to deteriorate. His girlfriend (Tanya) noticed that he was not as quick to answer questions at the pub quiz. He put his general lack of motivation down to stress at work and the threat of redundancy. Had it not been for a conversation Tanya had with his mum when she told her he was skipping football practice, Dennis would have carried on for a long time without a diagnosis. His mum too had noticed his lack of interest and lethargy and commented that it was unlike him not to want to go out and play football. Dennis admitted that he felt a bit out of sorts and his mum wondered whether he should see his GP. Dennis also said he had begun to experience pins and needles in his arms when he used his laptop and once or twice felt giddy when he got up from the chair. His mum suspected the worst and was glad when Dennis agreed to make a GP appointment.

The GP asked Dennis a few questions about his symptoms. He also took a blood sample. After he disclosed that his dad had MS, the GP decided to refer him to a neurologist at the local hospital.

The neurologist explained to Dennis that he would need to have a series of tests to investigate his symptoms. These included a lumbar puncture (LP, or spinal tap) to check the fluid in his spinal column as well as a magnetic resonance imaging (MRI) scan of his brain. He also explained that to confirm diagnosis he would need a number of electrical tests (evoked potential) to see what damage may have occurred to his nerve pathways.

After a few weeks Dennis was asked to go back and see the neurologist who confirmed test results showing signs of early onset MS.

The investigations carried out to diagnose MS vary, although MRI scans rather than the more traditional and invasive lumbar puncture are often performed. MRI scans are a very effective way of demonstrating changes in the brain caused by multiple sclerosis. It can show the neurologist clear signs of inflammation in the deep parts of the brain and spinal cord that are indicative of MS. However, the MRI brain scan test alone is not always conclusive since older people and those with high blood pressure and diabetes can also show inflammation in the brain which may imitate MS. It is necessary to do several investigations before confirming the diagnosis. It has also been known for a person with MS to have a normal MRI scan, as approximately 5 per cent of people with the condition do not have lesions in the brain; instead they may have lesions that do not show up on the MRI scan.

For a GP this is a very challenging situation, mainly because they may not encounter such patients very often. This makes it difficult to diagnose symptoms, especially as there is no single definitive test for MS. This accounts for the fact that many people remain undiagnosed for long periods.

DISEASE PROGRESSION AND TREATMENT

Disease progression and long-term outcomes are difficult to predict in MS. Positive outcomes are, moreover, more common in women, those who develop the disease early in life, those with a relapsing course and those who initially experienced few attacks (Pugliatti et al., 2002). Treatment attempts to improve function after an attack and prevent new attacks. There are 11 licensed treatments for MS, often referred to as disease-modifying therapies (DMTs). The drugs are largely available for people with relapsing, remitting MS and range from Tysabri, Lemtrada, oral therapies, to copaxone and the interferons. Large doses of steroids (methylprednisolone) are often used to treat relapses in order to reduce inflammation and are given intravenously in hospital or taken orally. Medications used to treat MS, while modestly effective, can have side effects and be poorly tolerated. Drug regimens such as interferon require a high level of compliance in order to achieve optimal efficiency (Freidel et al., 2015). In their study of the effects of interferon and nursing care, Freidel et al. found that in order to gain full benefit from disease-modifying therapies such as interferon β-1b, patients with MS needed to adhere to treatment in the long term. Their findings indicated that patients who rated nursing care as effective and valuable were more adherent to the drug regime. In other words, patients found it useful when nurses focused their attention on the individual problems identified by the patient. They also found that nursing care was valuable because they could trust the judgements of the nurse when providing information about the course of the disease. Despite the lack of therapeutic change in their condition following drug treatment, patients benefited from effective care that included information giving, telephone follow-up and close contact with nurses.

MEDICINAL CANNABIS AND MS

More recently, many people with MS are looking to complementary and alternative medicine (CAM) for answers to symptom control issues, despite a lack of sound evidence. One area of pain management that is becoming increasingly popular for people with MS is the use of medicinal cannabis for symptom control, specifically muscle spasticity. Specifically the use of cannabis for people with MS is symptomatic as MS is a neurological condition that gives rise to muscular pain and discomfort. Medicinal cannabis (sativex) can help to control the distress caused by muscle spasm and pain. It is available on the NHS although not in all parts of the country. Some GPs will prescribe it despite the cost and the lack of endorsement from NICE. It is available as a spray. The MS Society has published data on the rhetoric and reality of using cannabis on their website (www.mssociety.org.uk). Despite claims that cannabis is a natural drug its main ingredient is tetrahydrocannabinol (THC). THC is 'psychoactive', and can alter thinking and create hallucinations. People with MS who may have a family history of mental health problems (such as schizophrenia or bipolar disorder) are advised not to use cannabis as it can make the mental health symptoms worse. The other active ingredients in cannabis are cannabinoids (CBD), which have anti-inflammatory and antispasmodic properties. Here are some of the comments from patients with MS who have used cannabis.

NICKY'S STORY

66 Muscle spasms and stiffness cause my legs to clamp together, my arms to go rigid, and my body to fling itself backwards. Around four years ago I was able to try medicinal cannabis (sativex). It transformed my life. My neurologist and my GP submitted three requests for me to get sativex but each was unsuccessful. I'm now paying for sativex myself. It costs £500 a month. It's horrible for my kids to see me crying in pain. So I think the sacrifices have been worth it. 99

STEVE'S STORY

66 Spasticity causes excruciating cramps and rigidity in my legs. Sativex hugely improved my quality of life. But I have to pay for it myself. Over the past four years, I've only managed to buy seven months' worth. Cannabis isn't right for me but for those it helps, it should be made legal. 99

The clear message from the MS Society is that since cannabis is illegal there can be no full guidance about doses or quality; therefore, it is not possible to be confident that smoking cannabis is entirely safe and effective. This is why the MS Society is asking the UK government to review the current laws and make cannabis available for medicinal use in the treatment of muscular pain and spasms where other treatments have failed.

AUTOLOGOUS HAEMATOPOIETIC STEM CELL TRANSPLANTATION (HSCT)

Another area of palliative care treatment and symptom control for MS is autologous haematopoietic stem cell transplantation (HSCT), which involves the use of high doses of cancer chemotherapy drugs to wipe out harmful cells in the immune system. The patient's own stem cells are used to 'regrow' their immune system so that it no longer attacks myelin, thus reducing disease progression and preventing inflammation in the brain and spinal cord. The process involves taking a number of drugs to stimulate release of stem cells from the bone marrow into the blood stream. These cells are collected and kept frozen. The patient is then required to take chemotherapy drugs which either completely eliminate (myeloablative or high intensity chemotherapy) or partially eliminate (non-myeloablative or low-intensity chemotherapy) the bone marrow and immune system (Nash et al., 2017). Stem cell transplants carry risks and although all measures are taken to reduce these risks, clinical trials since 2001 have still had treatment-related death rates of one or two people in every hundred (Muraro et al., 2017). Current treatment methods for people with MS have favoured lower-intensity chemotherapy, which carries a lower risk of complications and death. This method results in the replenishment of the patient's immune system using his/her own stem cells. These cells then develop into the different types of cells found in the blood, including some cells which are part of the immune system. Recent research into the long-term outcomes of HSCT (Muraro et al., 2017; Nash et al., 2017) have reported on levels of disability in people with MS five years after receiving stem cell transplants. It is perhaps not suprising that HSCT take-up is quite low (Nash et al., 2017), especially when it is taken into account that the treatment involves enduring some distressing side effects from the drug.

PALLIATIVE CARE FOR PEOPLE WITH MS

Palliative care for people with MS is often not provided until the disease reaches the end of life stage. People with MS have symptom flare-ups and periods of remission when they feel independent and symptom free. This makes it difficult to provide consistent palliative care services, particularly when patients place great value on their ability to remain independent. However, when patients reach the palliative phase in their illness, palliative care can play a role in sustaining independence, rehabilitation and ensuring quality of life. This can occur through inpatient physiotherapy and occupational therapy (OT), both of which play a significant role in enabling people with MS to remain independent and develop self-management strategies to help optimise ADL functioning. Moreover, people with MS benefit from interventions made by occupational therapists who provide palliative care services, such as the provision of adaptations to the home. The OT services are focused on keeping the patient independent by using a range of equipment such as ramps for wheelchair access and grab rails to ease access to rooms and toilet facilities. In the palliative phase, the OT can facilitate the fitting of ceiling track hoists to aid moving and handling in and out of bed. Equipment is also provided to assist with a range of enhancements to ADL such as eating, drinking, washing, dressing and elimination needs.

One of the key features of the palliative care offered to people with MS is the focus on survivorship and wellbeing. The key message from groups like the MS Society internationally seems to be focused on the development of physical and psychological wellness through effective health promotion. Palliative care is focused on quality of life, and for many people with MS feeling good about themselves physically and psychologically is closely related to overall wellbeing (Wollin et al., 2006). Wellbeing is promoted in a variety of ways including health education and advice on issues such as nutrition, although at present, the role of nutrition is unclear, and MS therapy is not associated with any particular diet (Mowry et al., 2017). There is also help available on how to get support and treatment from professionals as well as help and information about medication and how to manage drug side effects as well as alternatives to conventional drugs. The following case study illustrates some of the key points about palliative care for people with MS.

CASE STUDY 4.2   SARAH

Sarah was a 66-year-old woman who lived in North Wales, diagnosed with MS at the age of 22. Sarah and her husband Eric had been married for 42 years with no children. In the initial years, Sarah was told that she had the progressive degenerative type of MS, which followed a pattern of remission and relapses. She spent much of her early life with MS getting used to periods when she felt very tired, and despite treatments and various remedies the fatigue became a difficult burden to bear. She also had problems with muscular weakness and spasticity. Just after she retired from work as a civil servant, Sarah suddenly became very unwell and she felt as if she had the flu. Her initial symptoms included a tremendous feeling of fatigue. She adapted to these symptoms initially although they did progressively become more severe. Over a period of one year she gradually began to lose her balance and this was followed by a lack of mobility. Over a two-year period she gradually became unable to walk. Sarah had always been underweight and over the initial few weeks of feeling ill her weight dropped to under 9 stone. Her GP paid a visit and confirmed her worst fears that it was in fact a severe flare-up of her MS. She was at least used to these over the years but since entering retirement she lived in fear and uncertainty about her health. Over a relatively short period Sarah's condition had deteriorated. Fortunately, with Eric's help and with assistance and support from friends, district nurses, Macmillan and Marie Curie nurses, Sarah was cared for at home. The district nurses called in a specialist MS nurse (Jenny) to advise them on how to provide the best care and she visited Sarah to help with her nursing assessment. Jenny listened to Sarah and asked her a lot of questions about her symptoms and what she felt they could do for her. Jenny checked the prescribed pain relief and also spent time talking to Eric and asking him how much support he was receiving. Eric received help from the community nursing team and

Marie Curie nurses provided a night sitting service once a week to enable him to get a good night's sleep. Jenny also advised Sarah to attend an MS therapy centre in Greater Manchester for specialist treatment and support. Sarah was interested, but was put off by the travelling. Over the next six months Sarah's condition deteriorated. The next visit by the district nurse prompted Sarah to discuss advance care planning.

Sarah's stated preference was to spend her last days at home with Eric and her Labrador dog Sheba. Sarah's main physical problems were anorexia, incontinence, weight loss, the development of pressure sores, swallowing difficulties and pain related to muscle spasticity. Despite the rapid decline in her physical condition she remained relatively alert and focused mentally. Sarah received palliative care from a range of community staff, including the GP, community physiotherapist and occupational therapists, social worker, speech therapist and community nursing staff (including the continence advisor nurse). They all played a part in enabling her to remain at home with a reasonable quality of life. The community nurses arranged for an NHS profile bed (with a pressure-relieving mattress) to be provided that enabled her to sit up. Ceiling hoists were fitted due to mobility issues and to help with moving and handling. In Sarah's case, her weight loss was quite extensive and Eric found he could move her about the bed by himself using a slide sheet. A commode was made available at the bedside. This was used in conjunction with a soft plastic bedpan that Sarah sometimes preferred to use. She eventually had an indwelling urinary catheter inserted towards the end of her life. Sarah was able to sit out of bed which she appreciated – having the dog at her feet and looking out of the window onto the countryside around her which she loved. Sarah was provided with oxygen via a nasal cannula (24%) as her breathing became more laboured especially as a result of the chest infection she developed towards the end of her life. She developed a chest infection and refused antibiotics, as she was aware that she was near the end of life. Sarah died in the early hours of the morning three months after her initial flu symptoms. She remained mentally competent most of the time. Eric described it as a 'good death'.

Sarah's case study highlights a number of physical problems that occur throughout the course of the disease that remain very relevant at the end of life. One of these, which is susceptible to palliative care treatment, is spasticity of the muscles (Embrey, 2009; Edwards et al., 2008). It is one of the most distressing symptoms of MS and requires the use of a range of muscle relaxants such as buscapan and antispasmodics such as baclofen, and drugs such as diazepam to treat muscular spasms that occur at night. Sarah's GP prescribed a range of drugs that could be used as required that included baclofen, gabapentin steroids and a range of pain killers non-opiates such as tramadol and morphine (MST). NICE guidance (2014) on the use of antispasmodics recommends the use of baclofen or gabapentin as first-line drug treatments to treat spasticity in MS depending on contraindications and the person's comorbidities and preferences. Gabapentin is a drug used in the treatment of neuropathic pain in multiple sclerosis. It is specifically used to treat pain caused by the effects of MS, such as trigeminal neuralgia or abnormal sensations (dysaesthesia), such as burning or pins and needles. It is also used for the treatment of spasticity although one of its side effects is fatigue. NICE guidance (2014) suggests that if the person with MS cannot tolerate one of these drugs, consider switching to other antispasmodic drugs such as tizanidine or dantrolene as a second-line option to treat spasticity. A third option is the use of benzodiazepines.

In some cases, patients can (although Sarah did not) have antispasmodic drugs intrathecally via a pump in order to ensure therapeutic levels are maintained. Sarah's GP, Bob, was aware of her MS and had prescribed antispasmodics for many years previously, he was aware of her wishes and ensured that she had a regular prescription.

NICE GUIDANCE ON SYMPTOM MANAGEMENT

- People with MS should have tried the drug at an optimal dose, or the maximum dose they can tolerate. Moreover, the drug should be discontinued if there is no benefit at the maximum tolerated dose.
- Once the optimal dose has been reached, the patient needs to have all their medication reviewed at least annually.
- Drugs used to control spasticity – i.e. baclofen or gabapentin – should be used as first-line drugs to treat spasticity in MS depending on contraindications and the person's comorbidities and preferences. If the person with MS cannot tolerate one of these drugs, consider switching to the other.
- Drugs such as tizanidine or dantrolene should be used as second-line options to treat spasticity in people with MS.
- Benzodiazepines should be considered as a third-line option to treat spasticity in MS. Prescribing physicians need to be aware of their potential benefit in treating nocturnal spasms.
- Should symptoms of spasticity not be managed with any of the stated pharmacological treatments, the patient should be referred to specialist spasticity services.

NICE guidance (2014) on the management of symptoms does not endorse the use of medicinal cannabis (sativex) because it is not cost effective. The guidance makes it clear that individual GPs can make their own decisions about its cost and effectiveness.

NON-PHARMACOLOGICAL FORMS OF TREATMENT

The control of muscle stiffness for Sarah was a key symptom and was focused on by the nurses who carried out active and passive leg exercises (as Eric did in their absence), physical movement was supported by the physiotherapist, a key contributor to the palliative care team (Holland et al., 2011). The overarching problem of muscle spasm and muscle pain is often a very common problem (Rosti-Otajarv and Hamalainen, 2011) and patients like Sarah use their own strategies to relieve stiffness such as heat pads, and warm baths so it's important to listen and act on the patient and carer's advice as healthcare professionals

(Malcolmson et al., 2008). Closely related to muscle management is insomnia as the reason for lack of sleep is often muscle spasm. The MS Society UK produces some very useful advice on how to manage insomnia that includes doing more during the day and basic exercises. Together Sarah and Eric ensured that they had a routine: a set time to wake up and to go to bed, regular meal times, lots of rest and some activity.

Management of continence was a key issue for Sarah as well as many patients with MS at the end of life. Finding and utilising appropriate continence aids can improve quality of life and the continence advisor was beneficial in helping to assess Sarah's individual needs. Initially Sarah was reluctant to have an indwelling urinary catheter because of the risk of infection in the long term. This was discussed during the session on advanced care planning and the nurses persuaded Sarah of the need to stay continent by having an indwelling urinary catheter inserted towards the end of her life in order to prevent the complications of pressure ulcers and to prevent loss of dignity. Consideration was given to having a suprapubic catheter surgically inserted to prevent infection, in order to avoid the problem of bypassing of urine around the catheter. Sarah did not wish to have that type of catheter and wanted minimal invasive medical intervention. A further physical challenge to optimising palliative care was maintaining skin integrity. Skin care and the prevention of decubitus ulcers in patients towards the end of life is a prime consideration in terms of quality of life. Physical challenges often centre on the prevention and management of the consequences of problems such as pressure ulcers that can add to disability.

This is an issue highlighted in the NICE guidelines. Infections (especially respiratory and urinary tract infection) are a constant threat to quality of life especially in the advanced stages of the disease (NICE, 2003). The guidelines highlight the need for attention to be given to hygiene (both person and caregiver, with a focus on hand washing when emptying catheters and if self-catheterisation is used (NICE, 2003). In Sarah's case, Eric was such a diligent and meticulous caregiver that options such as self-catheterisation were not required. Sarah used a Silastic indwelling urinary catheter with a short leg bag at night and a long bag during the day when able to sit out of bed. Infection is a major issue depending on the person's level of mobility; the more disabled people become, the greater the risk of infection. Many people with MS lose the ability to walk before death, 90 per cent are capable of independent walking at 10 years from onset, and 75 per cent at 15 years (Rossier and Wade, 2002).

Apart from the physical challenges, there are numerous psychosocial aspects to living with MS that nurses and healthcare professionals need to be aware of in order to provide optimal care (Patten and Metz, 2002). The psychological issues can and do begin with the diagnosis and the transition to living with MS, coping with the symptoms, the relapses and the treatment (Malcomson et al., 2008). Depression and suicide are more common in people with MS than other neurological conditions (Royal College of Physicians, 2011). This is related to the roller coaster type illness trajectory which accompanies MS, with some patients having no active symptoms for years yet knowing they may reoccur, living in a cognitive and emotional climate of uncertainty about remission and relapse times. Specialist nurses who work with people with MS express empathy, compassion and understanding of the disease but remain focused on keeping the patient in control as much as possible to retain autonomy (De Broe et al., 2001). Clearly, the focus of the nurse is on the patient, although palliative care practitioners will recognise the importance of supporting caregivers who may often feel despair and frustration towards the patient, especially when employment is affected and financial stability becomes an issue (McKeown et al., 2003). Patients with MS also express concern about the level of social care provided by statutory bodies as limited resources and cutbacks can mean more financial hardship for families and individuals (Chang et al., 2002).

PALLIATIVE CARE AT THE END OF LIFE FOR PEOPLE WITH MS

In relation to palliative care at the end of life, illness progression and cause of death are invariably related to the consequences of the disease, with infection being a major cause of mortality at the end of life (Tsang and Macdonell, 2011). The patient's prognosis is dependent on a number of factors, namely: gender, age, the subtype of the disease and the early onset of symptoms as well as the extent of the individual's disability (Ontaneda et al., 2017). One of the key features of MS, as illustrated by Sarah's case study, was the prolonged uncertainty that periods of remission can create. For many patients and their partners and caregivers, the experience of MS is shrouded in uncertainty. This can create a false sense of security and hope that the disease itself has burnt out. This may perhaps help to explain the irritation and severe frustration that is often reported by people with MS. The previous case study provides an illustration of one woman's experience of living with and dying from the progressive degenerative type of MS. There are several major nursing challenges to the provision of effective palliative care for people like Sarah at the end of life. Broadly, these challenges can be considered as physical, psychological and social (Freidel et al., 2015). One of the key symptoms experienced by many patients with MS is fatigue (Motl al., 2017).

Fatigue may be described as an extreme form of tiredness in which the lethargy has a pervading effect on the individual's ability to carry out activities of daily living (ADL) and impacts on their emotional wellbeing. Motl et al. (2017) refer to the term 'wellness' when considering a range of symptoms associated with fatigue. One of the key physical challenges with Sarah was nutrition since her weight loss impacted on her risk of developing a pressure ulcer. The state of knowledge regarding diet and MS is limited and no single type of diet has demonstrated any proven

effects on the prevention of symptom development (Lorenz et al., 2008). It is important in the palliative phase of Sarah's illness to refer her to the dietician and speech
therapist for advice on the best diet, means of hydration and ways to promote
swallowing (Motl et al., 2017).

In terms of nutrition, a major challenge for people with advanced MS like
Sarah was swallowing. Dysphagia represents a safety issue due to problems of
choking and often requires food to be purified or made into a soft small bolus
for easier digestion. One of the key contributors to the multidisciplinary palliative care team is the speech and language therapist (SLT). The speech therapist
and dietician played a key role in advising the district nurses about her diet;
little and often, small amounts of food to be cooked by Eric, food made easier
to swallow by the use of a blender, crème freche, ice cream, bananas, fruit and
her favourite dish lasagne, followed by chocolate. The speech therapist recommended that if, and when, it became impossible for Sarah to swallow, a
nasogastric tube or percutaneous endoscopic gastronomy (PEG), tube feeding,
could be used. The latter involves inserting a tube into the stomach and suturing
the tube into the abdominal wall. Neither of these were acceptable to Sarah and
while quite invasive, PEG tubes are often preferred to a nasogastric tube that is
visible and very uncomfortable. In her advance care planning, Sarah stipulated
that she was against artificial forms of feeding on the basis that she lost her
dignity. An even more invasive form of feeding is parenteral feeding, where
patients are fed with special dietary fluid directly into the vein, although this
form of feeding is often not preferred by patients unless absolutely necessary as
it limits their mobility. In all cases of feeding it is important that nurses ensure
that the patient has good oral hygiene and where possible is encouraged to feed
themselves even if it is small amounts of fluid or sucking ice cubes to refresh the
mouth. There is no substitute for eating food that has been selected and preferred by the patient.

Spirituality is an area not touched on in the case study, partly because it was not
an issue that came up between Sarah, Eric and the palliative care team. Spiritual
care is often discussed in relation to end of life, although few nurses would claim
to have a thorough knowledge of what spiritual care involves in a secular society
(Cobb et al., 2012). Should the patient state a particular religious orientation, they
may be offered the services of a member of the hospital/hospice spiritual care team.
For a more in-depth discussion of spiritual care see Chapter 9.

SUPPORT FOR CAREGIVERS

Central to effective palliative care at the end of life is emotional and practical
support for caregivers (Costello, 2017). In the case study Eric, Sarah's husband, received a range of support from the community nurses, the local MS
Society group, through online contact, local groups, as well as friends and
ex-work colleagues.

CASE STUDY 4.3   ERIC'S STORY (CASE STUDY 4.2 CONTINUED)

I was not terribly shocked by the news that Sarah's MS had become much worse. In many ways I had been anticipating this event for many years. Strangely enough, the support we received from the local MS group made us aware that this time would come. That does not mean to say that it was not a distressing and worrying time. At first I busied myself with making changes to the house to accommodate Sarah's loss of independence. Like many people with MS this is a big issue. I moved the bed downstairs and the community nurses arranged for a commode which she hated but put up with because I made sure I looked after it. I was surprised by the suddenness of the change, even though we had talked about it in the local support group. Somehow, you can never be fully prepared. Looking back, I was glad of having lots to do. I had been retired two years and I had my wood turning and my workshop which I used to retire to when I wanted time alone. On reflection, I feel as if I was given a lot of support and it was always available to me if I needed it. I was made aware that a lot of couples split up after a few years of living with MS. I suppose I was lucky in that I knew what I was getting into with Sarah as she was diagnosed before we married. I understood MS and we had a good life and we helped each other, it was not one way traffic, although towards the end I was having to do a lot. Most of the support I received came from the local support group. People would phone me up and we would chat together with Sarah on speaker. I had a lot of discussions online which was helpful. The nurses were good but I knew their time was limited so I always tried to let them know I was OK and they should get on with their work. Our biggest challenge (or mine) was during the night when I could hear Sarah groaning with the pain and she needed turning because she was getting sore. I was worried about her getting pressure sores and made it my mission to prevent this, although she did have small ones on each ankle and redness on her hips and bottom. This caused Sheba, who slept by her bed, to start barking and we ended up having tea and talking for a while after. Afterwards I found it hard to get back to sleep and the next day I was physically and mentally tired and would fall asleep and nap. Sarah tried not to disturb me and let me rest even when she needed me, like the time she had an accident because she let me sleep during the day. We argued about this type of thing. Eventually we got night sitters to come in, which was a great help as I could go out, have a couple of beers, get her ready for bed and I could get a good night's sleep. We were lucky in that we had a good team of nurses and others like the physio who helped Sarah at the end to get her breathing sorted. Sarah was the star. She was her usual thoughtful, kind and considerate self and although we had a plan for the end, it was not easy and I heard her shed a few tears alone. We both shared a lot of truths about the end but made sure not to dwell on it. The last week, I did not sleep much. We were both tired, her chest was bad but the morphine helped a lot and I was happy to give her sips of water to moisten her lips and do all the things the nurses did. It gave me something to do and helped me to feel wanted. I look back and consider myself lucky to have had such a great wife and I feel slightly proud that I contributed to what I call a 'good death', if there is such a thing.

CONCLUSION

This chapter has described the key symptoms and varied treatments used to improve the quality of life for people who have MS. Moreover, the chapter has focused on the provision of palliative care for people with MS at intermittent stages during the illness and at the end of life. It has been acknowledged that the provision of quality palliative care takes into account the unpredictable nature of the condition. In general, most people with MS and other non-cancer conditions prefer to die at home, as the case study of Sarah showed. It is clear, however, that for many reasons, such as the vulnerability of the caregiver, this is not always possible. The case studies illustrate the complexity of multiple sclerosis and its diagnosis, and the role of palliative care before the onset of advanced disease and in providing end of life care. Moreover, the chapter situated the importance of the role of palliative care in meeting the individual needs of the patient and providing emotional support for the caregiver. Palliative care can be provided as short-term care or can encompass more long-term provision to incorporate end of life care.

A version of this chapter was published in the *International Journal of Palliative Nursing,* Volume 23, Issue 10, 474–483. Under the title 'Preserving the independence of people living with multiple sclerosis towards the end of life' with kind permission of SAGE Publications Ltd.

REFERENCES

Alonso, A, Jick, S., Olek, M. and Hernín, M. (2007) 'Incidence of multiple sclerosis in the United Kingdom.' *Journal of Neurology, 254*: 1736–41.

Chang, C.H., Cell, D., Fernandez, O., Lugue, G. et al. (2002) 'Quality of life in multiple sclerosis patients in Spain.' *Multiple Sclerosis,* 8: 527–31.

Cobb, M.R., Puchalski, C.M. and Rumbold B. (2012) *Oxford Textbook of Spirituality in Healthcare.* Oxford University Press.

Costello, J. (2017) 'The role of informal caregivers at the end of life: providing support through advance care planning.' *International Journal of Palliative Nursing, 23* (2): 60–5.

De Broe, S., Christopher, F. and Waugh N. (2001) 'The role of specialist nurses in multiple sclerosis: a rapid and systematic review.' *Health Technology Assessment,* 5: 1–52.

Edwards, R.G., Barlow, J.H. and Turner, A.P. (2008) 'Experiences of diagnosis and treatment among people with multiple sclerosis'. *Journal of Evaluation in Clinical Practice,* 14: 460–4.

Embrey, N. (2009) 'Exploring the lived experience of palliative care for people with MS, 3: Group support'. *British Journal of Neuroscience Nursing.* 5: 402–8.

Freidel, M., Ortler, S., Fuchs, A., Seibert, S. and Schuh, K. (2015) 'Acceptance of the Extracare Program by beta interferon-treated patients with multiple sclerosis.' *Journal of Neuroscience Nursing, 47* (1): E31–9.

Holland, N.J., Schneider, D.M., Rapp, R. and Kalb, R.C. (2011) 'Meeting the needs of people with primary progressive MS, their families and the health care community.' *International Journal of MS Care, 13*: 65–74.

Lorenz, K.A., Lynn S.M., Dy, S.M., Shugarman, L.R. et al. (2008) 'Evidence for improving palliative care at the end of life: a systematic review.' *Annals of Internal Medicine, 148* (2): 147–59.

Malcolmson, K.S., Lowe-Strong, A.S. and Dunwoody, L. (2008) 'What can we learn from the personal insights of individuals living and coping with multiple sclerosis?' *Disability and Rehabilitation, 30*: 662–74.

McKeown, L.P., Porter-Armstrong, A.P. and Baxter, G.D. (2003) 'The needs and experiences of caregivers of individuals with MS: a systematic review'. *Clinical Rehabilitation, 17*: 234–48.

Methley, A.M., Chew-Graham, C. and Campbell, S. (2014) 'Experiences of UK health related care services for people with multiple sclerosis: a systematic narrative review.' *Health Expectations, 18* (6): 1844–55.

Motl, R.W., Mowry, E.M., Ehde, D.M., LaRocca, N.G. et al. (2017) 'Wellness and multiple sclerosis: the National MS Society establishes a wellness research working group and research priorities.' *Multiple Sclerosis*. doi: 10.1177/1352458516687404

MS Society (2017) Cannabis and MS. www.mssociety.org.uk/cannabis-and-ms, accessed 8 September 2017.

Muraro, P., Pasquini, M., Atkins, H.L., Bowen, J.D. et al. (2017) 'Long-term outcomes after autologous hematopoietic stem cell transplantation for multiple sclerosis.' *JAMA Neurology*. doi: 10.1001/jamaneurol.2016.5867

Nash, M.J., Frank, D.N. and Friedman, J.E. (2017) 'Early Microbes Modify Immune System Development and Metabolic Homeostasis – The "Restaurant" Hypothesis Revisited'. *Frontiers in Endocrinology*. doi.org/10.3389/fendo.2017.00349 (accessed July 2018).

NICE (2003) *Multiple Sclerosis: National Clinical Guidelines for Diagnosis and Management in Primary and Secondary Care*. CG8. London: NICE.

NICE (2014) *Multiple Sclerosis in Adults: Management*. CG186. London: NICE.

Ontaneda, D., Thompson, A.J., Fox, R.J. and Cohen, J.A. (2017) 'Progressive multiple sclerosis: prospects for disease therapy, repair, and restoration of function.' *The Lancet, 389* (10076): 1357–66.

Patten, S.B. and Metz, L.M. (2002) 'Hopelessness ratings in relapsing remitting and secondary progressive multiple sclerosis.' *International Journal of Psychiatry Medicine, 32*, 155–65.

Pugliatti, M., Sotgiu, S. and Rosati G. (2002) 'The worldwide prevalence of multiple sclerosis.' *Clinical Neurological Neurosurgery, 104*, 3, 182–91.

Rossier, P. and Wade, D.T. (2002) 'The Guy's Disability Neurological Scale in patients with multiple sclerosis: a clinical evaluation of its reliability and validity.' *Clinical Rehabilitation, 16* (1): 75–9.

Rosti-Otajarv, E.M. and Hamalainen, P.I. (2011) 'Neuropsychological rehabilitation for multiple sclerosis.' *Cochrane Database of Systematic Reviews, 11*. doi:1002/14651858. cd009131.pub2

Royal College of Physicians (2011) *The National Audit of Services for People with MS*. London: Royal College of Physicians.

Solomon, A.J. and Corboy, J.R. (2017) 'The tension between early diagnosis and misdiagnosis of multiple sclerosis.' *Nature Reviews Neurology*. doi:10.1038/nrneurol.2017.106

Tsang, B.K. and Macdonell, R. (2011) 'Multiple sclerosis—diagnosis, management and prognosis.' *Aust Fam Physician, 40*(12): 948–55.

Wollin, J.A., Yates, P.M. and Kristjanson, L.J. (2006) 'Supportive and palliative care needs identified by multiple sclerosis patients and their families.' *International Journal of Palliative Nursing, 12* (1): 20–6.

FURTHER READING

Edmonds, P., Hart, S. and Gao, W. (2010) 'Palliative care for people severely affected by multiple sclerosis: evaluation of a novel palliative care service.' *Multiple Sclerosis*, 16 (5): 627–36.

Giesser, B.S. (ed.) (2016) *Primer on Multiple Sclerosis*. 2nd ed. Oxford: Oxford University Press.

Healthline (2018) *Understanding Multiple Sclerosis (MS)*. Available at www.healthline.com/health/multiple-sclerosis, accessed April 2018.

National MS Society (2018) *What Is MS?* Available at www.nationalmssociety.org/What-is-MS, accessed April 2018.

Palliative Care Australia (2018) *National Palliative Care Standards*. 5th ed. Available at http://palliativecare.org.au/standards, accessed April 2018.

Strupp, J., Groebe, B., Knies, A., Mai, M., Voltz, R. and Golla, H. (2018) 'Evaluation of a palliative and hospice care telephone hotline for patients severely affected by multiple sclerosis and their caregivers.' *European Journal of Neurology*, 24 (12): 1518–24.

5

PATIENTS WITH END STAGE RENAL FAILURE

SUSAN HEATLEY

LEARNING OUTCOMES

- Describe the pathophysiology of renal disease
- Explain the stages of the disease and common forms of treatment
- Give an account of the nursing care for patients with end stage renal disease
- Provide the patient and nurse's perspective on renal disease

INTRODUCTION

This chapter focuses on people with chronic kidney disease (CKD), a condition that over time results in end stage renal disease (ESRD). CKD is not as common as other long-term conditions, such as heart disease, respiratory disease and cancer, but worldwide over two million individuals receive renal replacement therapy in the form of dialysis (Liyanage, 2015). The first section provides background information and a review of the pathophysiology of the disease. It also includes a focus on different forms of treatment that is often time-consuming but lifesaving. The experience of providing care in the palliative stage of the disease is considered from the nurse's perspective, and finally a living account of the disease is provided by a patient with many years' experience of renal dialysis.

BACKGROUND

In the UK it has been well established that the number of patients receiving dialysis is increasing, with poor outcomes and high cost. Despite medical advances, many patients who reach end stage renal disease (ESRD) and require dialysis therapy die each year (Cohen et al., 2006). Studies have shown that symptom burden in patients undergoing dialysis therapy is as high as that of cancer patients (Saini et al., 2006; Davison, 2010). In the UK the average lifespan of patients starting dialysis over the age of 65 with one or more comorbidities is two years (Murtagh et al., 2006). It is becoming more evident that a seamless structure of supportive care incorporating holistic components of physical care, psychological care, social care and spiritual care is needed as renal patients embark on their journey from diagnosis to death (Cohen et al., 2006). This has forced a paradigm shift in nephrology towards a focus on palliative and end of life care.

PATHOPHYSIOLOGY

CKD is a progressive, irreversible deterioration in renal function in which the body's ability to maintain metabolic and fluid and electrolyte balance fails, resulting in uraemia (retention of urea and other nitrogenous wastes in the blood). As renal function declines, the end products of protein metabolism (which are normally excreted in urine) accumulate in the blood, uraemia develops and adversely affects every system in the body. The greater the build-up of waste products results in the patient developing severe signs and symptoms, which include neurologic weakness, fatigue, confusion, restless legs, dry flaky skin, pruritus, thinning hair, cardiovascular hypertension, oedema, pericardial friction rub, pericarditis, shortness of breath, metallic taste, anorexia, nausea and vomiting, constipation or diarrhoea, anaemia, decreased libido, muscle cramps and bone pain.

CKD may be caused by systemic diseases, such as diabetes mellitus (leading cause); hypertension; chronic glomerulonephritis; pyelonephritis (inflammation of the renal pelvis); obstruction of the urinary tract; hereditary lesions, as in polycystic kidney disease; vascular disorders; infections; medications; or toxic agents. Comorbid conditions that develop during CKD contribute to high morbidity and mortality among patients with CKD. Dialysis or kidney transplantation eventually becomes necessary for patient survival.

DIALYSIS

Dialysis, an artificial replacement for lost kidney function, is used to treat stage 5 CKD (see Table 5.1) and is normally initiated when there is evidence of uraemia. Uraemia equates to CKD stage 5 or an estimated glomerular filtration rate (eGFR) <15 ml/minute.

Table 5.1   Stages of CKD

Stage	Description	eGFR ml/min
1	Slight kidney disease	90 or above
2	Mild decrease in kidney function	60–89
3	Moderate decrease in kidney function	30–59
4	Severe decrease in kidney function	15–29
5	Kidney failure requiring dialysis	Less than 15

DIALYSIS THERAPIES

Making the decision on which form of dialysis to choose is complex because it involves major changes in one's lifestyle and dependence on a treatment without which life would cease (Muringai et al., 2008). There are two types of dialysis treatment: haemodialysis and peritoneal dialysis. In order to start haemodialysis patients have vascular access surgery to create an arteriovenous fistula (AVF) which is the creation of a link between an artery and a vein in the arm (see Figure 5.1). Dialysis usually takes place in a haemodialysis unit three times a week, for four hours on each occasion. It involves a patient's blood being pumped from the fistula through tubing to a haemodialysis machine. The machine acts like a kidney, filtering waste products from the blood before returning it to the patient.

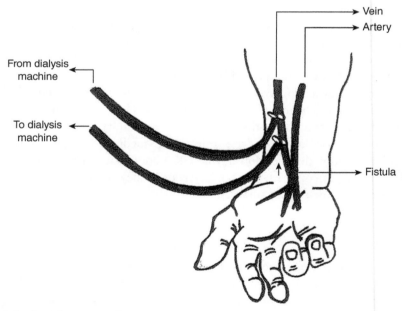

Figure 5.1   Arteriovenous fistula

Source: Original drawing by Betty Deway

Patients undergoing hospital haemodialysis tend to receive the minimal hours of dialysis treatment (4 hours) three times a week; studies have shown a strong and consistent association with lower dialysis times with increased mortality and symptom burden. Intradialytic symptoms (those relating to the dialysis procedure) are common and include hypotension, cramps, nausea and vomiting, and pruritis. In addition, post-haemodialysis hypotension and a 'washed out' feeling lasting up to 24 hours are also common. Patients undergoing hospital haemodialysis endure additional time travelling to and from the dialysis unit, waiting to be attached to the machine, and waiting for their needle sites to stop bleeding at the end of treatment.

PERITONEAL DIALYSIS

Other patients are managed on peritoneal dialysis (PD), where a catheter is placed in the peritoneum and dialysis fluid is entered into the patient's peritoneal cavity (the inner 'belly'), which is covered by a thin membrane containing many small blood vessels. Toxins from the blood diffuse into the peritoneal cavity across the peritoneal membrane. The advantage of peritoneal dialysis is that the patient can remain active while the dialysis is proceeding. This is known as continuous ambulatory peritoneal dialysis (CAPD) and must be carried out four times a day (see Figure 5.2). Peritoneal dialysis can also be carried out overnight, forgoing the need to carry out the dialysis procedure four times a day.

PD has several advantages as well as limitations. Unlike haemodialysis, PD delivers a steady-state treatment avoiding wide fluctuations of fluid volume and solutes. In addition, PD provides flexible schedules (unlike fixed hospital haemodialysis shifts), therefore providing opportunities to work, travel and participate in daytime activities for patients.

Despite some advantages of PD, there are several drawbacks (see Table 5.2). PD being a continuous therapy with no 'off' days may be inconvenient and can cause fatigue and burnout of patients and families. Some patients may have concern with body image resulting from the presence of catheter and fluid in the abdomen. Moreover, there are various complications associated with PD which include infections (peritonitis, exit site and tunnel), dialysate protein loss, metabolic complications from dialysate glucose absorption and weight gain.

Like peritoneal dialysis, haemodialysis can be carried out in the home by patients, with some potential clinical benefits compared to hospital-based haemodialysis, including improved survival, quality of life and health system costs (Rygh et al., 2012). As a result, nephrologists believe home dialysis modalities should constitute a larger proportion of patients than is currently the case (Wilkie, 2011). Despite these perceptions, hospital-based haemodialysis remains the predominant form of dialysis treatment in the UK (Wilkie, 2011).

Although dialysis is often seen as a requirement to prolong life, without which people will die, it is an arduous therapy known to shorten life (United States Renal Data System, 2015). Patients on dialysis often experience a multitude of symptoms

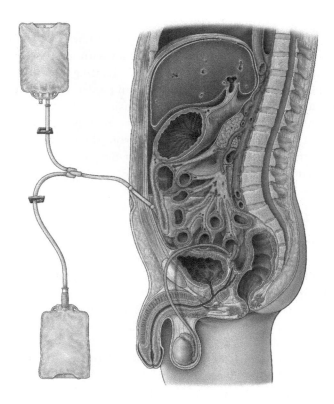

Figure 5.2   Peritoneal dialysis

Source: Science Photo Library

resulting from their renal disease, dietary and fluid restrictions and dialysis treatment. It also necessitates extensive changes in lifestyle that impact on many aspects
of life and challenge the ability of patients to maintain an acceptable quality of life
(Jablonski, 2007).

Table 5.2   Disadvantages/side effects of peritoneal dialysis

Effect/Outcome	Source/Remedy
Constipation	Caused by dialysis drying out the bowel
Bloating	Caused by fluid in the abdomen
Permanent catheter	Affects body image as protrudes from abdomen
Peritonitis	So need to be ultra-careful with hygiene
Dressing changes	Need to do every time you have a bath or shower
Changes to diet	Need low salt and low phosphate diet
Treatment every day	Either 4 exchanges per day or overnight each night
Storage	Large number of boxes of fluid and other equipment
Phosphate binders	Need to be taken with every meal

PATIENT PERCEPTIONS AND EXPERIENCES OF THEIR DISEASE AND TREATMENTS

Chronic kidney disease is a multifaceted problem, having both physical and psychological connotations for the patient. Patients on dialysis are in a situation of wretched dependence on a machine, a procedure and a group of qualified medical/nursing professionals for the rest of his/her life (Reichsman and Levy, 1972). Despite its lifesaving qualities, dialysis treatment is time-consuming, intrusive and can be burdensome for some patients (Polaschek, 2003). Compared with the general population, dialysis patients consistently perceive themselves as having a poor health-related quality of life (HRQL), in particular in the dimension of physical functioning (Finkelstein et al., 2009). Reduced physical functioning compromises employment opportunities and participation in social and leisure activities.

Some studies suggest that dialysis patients who display negative perceptions of their illness have an increased risk of depression (Cvengros et al., 2005). Perceiving CKD as a negative intrusion into lifestyle is more likely to be associated with poorer treatment compliance and higher symptom burden (Kutner et al., 2009). However, adherence to dialysis regimes does not always relieve the physiological complications of CKD for all patients, with some continuing to experience the distressing physical symptoms of their disease. Patients begin to realise that the technology of dialysis minimises some of the physical symptoms but does not prevent further deterioration in their physical health (Polascheck, 2003).

Research carried out on patients' experience of CKD on dialysis offers a valuable and interesting insight into a patient's perceptions and experience of illness and treatment (Trimmers et al., 2008). A significant number of patients associate their disease and dialysis treatments with being a burden, demanding, life restricting, painful, time consuming; feelings of powerlessness, feebleness, exhaustion and suffering are also commonly expressed by some patients.

The patient's whole life situation is turned upside down with chronic kidney disease when they are confronted with the forced change to start haemodialysis treatment. The psychosocial adjustment of patients to a programme of dialysis treatment is influenced positively or negatively by their personality and lifestyle. A key influence on their experience of the disease is the support they receive from their renal team and their families. Paul's story provides an insight into his life on hospital haemodialysis:

66 I was in my early twenties when I was started on dialysis treatment at my local dialysis centre and naturally I found the change of lifestyle traumatic. My friends would be out every weekend, but that all had to stop for me. Due to the renal disease and dialysis treatment I can now no longer work, although I did try to return to work but the change in my energy levels and the symptoms I was experiencing made working impossible. I often feel

down in the dumps and shattered after my dialysis and just want to lie down and go to sleep. I feel my family have missed out on so much because I'm not able to do normal everyday things.

Paul, patient with CKD

Sandra's story provides a slightly different insight into hospital dialysis

When I started on dialysis at the renal unit I was feeling pretty unwell, scared and not too sure what to expect. After a few sessions I began to feel a little better and I found I was enjoying going to the unit three times a week because I could meet other patients and the staff looked after me very well. Going three days a week means I can still have four days off and spend time with my family although sometimes dialysis makes me feel tired, but you just get on with it.

Sandra, patient with CKD

The literature suggests that home dialysis is more clinically effective and cheaper than haemodialysis in hospital (Robinson et al., 2016). Home dialysis is growing in popularity due to the flexibility and benefits it brings to patients' lives. Both peritoneal dialysis and haemodialysis can be performed by the patient in their own home. Patients who choose or are able to carry out home dialysis have more free time and gain a deeper understanding of their health conditions, which often leads to less fear and depression and a more positive outlook on the future (Blagg, 2008).

Irene's story provides us with a different perspective on dialysis treatments when carried out in the home:

From lying in the hospital three days a week with that haemodialysis and being ill and in bad shape and everything, when I changed to doing my dialysis at home it was quite a different everyday life for me. I now see how much better I am, and how much better I function in everyday life … you can utilise the day better; not a problem to be fully employed, I am enjoying being in control of my illness and my life in general.

Irene, patient with CKD

NURSE PERCEPTIONS

Work in dialysis centres is marked by intensive and long-term contact with chronically ill patients who are frequently frustrated or depressive (Bilgic et al., 2007). This confrontation with suffering and death is very demanding for the nursing/medical staff in dialysis centres (Ashker et al., 2012). Dialysis nurses have a special relationship with their patients; due to the nature of long-term dialysis, relationships are usually forged after a long association of months and in some cases many years. Jenkins et al. (2002) suggest that a good nurse–patient relationship in a dialysis setting is essential to meet the clinical, psychological and social needs of the patient in order to optimise treatment.

As well as the technical aspects of dialysis care, other roles of the dialysis nurse include caregiver, advocate, educator, facilitator and mentor. The literature offers both positive and negative aspects of renal nurses' perceptions on working with patients undergoing hospital dialysis. Helen is a renal nurse working in a hospital-based haemodialysis centre. She says:

> As renal nurses we are a big part of our patients' lives as we are their 'lifeline' in providing dialysis. I believe that creating an environment of comfort and feeling at home is an important part of what we do. As renal nurses, we get to assist the patient with attempting to achieve the highest quality of life they can attain, despite having a life-limiting condition which requires dialysis treatment three times a week. It's also rewarding to help patients to stay healthy on dialysis. I feel I am very lucky to have a job where I get to know the patients extremely well and build up long-term relationships sharing their personal life stories.
>
> Helen, renal nurse

However, the literature suggests that nurses working in hospital dialysis units have high levels of emotional exhaustion linked to the stress of the job (Hayes et al., 2015). In addition, the context of prolonged relationships with patients in the haemodialysis environment can over time become emotionally draining and a source of stress, particularly when patients die. Traditionally, nurses are encouraged to provide a stoic persona in the face of emotional pressures in the workplace. However, objective stoicism is difficult when close personal relationships are formed with patients (Diefendorff et al., 2011).

Wendy, a hospital haemodialysis nurse, explains:

> I have worked at the hospital dialysis unit for seven years now and I can say I am really not enjoying it too much. The work is repetitive and you see the same patients three times a week indefinitely. You do develop relationships with patients but this can be both good and not so good relationships. Then there is all the technical stuff that you have to be proficient at, not to mention all the moving and cleaning of the dialysis machines. Every day is the same.
>
> Wendy, haemodialysis nurse

CASE STUDY 5.1   SIVA: A PATIENT'S EXPERIENCE OF DIALYSIS

This section begins by looking at renal disease from the patient Siva's perspective, focusing largely on the experience of a patient being on renal dialysis and how this impacts on them physically and emotionally. It also considers the influence of treatment on quality of life.

My first experience of dialysis came about as a result of developing renal failure (see Chapter 1), and I was admitted to a high dependency unit. I was informed, following a kidney biopsy, that the damage to my kidneys was permanent and I was put on haemodialysis. In order to provide access for the dialysis I had a femoral line inserted, which I hated. A femoral line is only used for short periods before being replaced. I was anxious for an alternative, which came in the form of a permacath. A permacath is a piece of plastic tubing – very similar to a jugular catheter – and is used in exactly the same way for haemodialysis. The permacath has a cuff that holds the catheter in place and acts as a barrier to infection. The cuff is underneath the skin and cannot be seen.

I was told that in the future, I would have a fistula formed. Overall, I found the dialysis regime quite exhausting. To the amazement of the medical staff, I regained some kidney function and a month later I was discharged without dialysis and the permacath was removed. It is difficult to describe how overjoyed I was by this news.

A year later, at a routine follow-up clinic, high amounts of protein were discovered in my urine. A kidney biopsy revealed that my kidneys were once again deteriorating and I would need further dialysis. The news was most upsetting and I can remember the depression I felt.

IMPACT OF TREATMENT

Further haemodialysis meant travelling to hospital three times a week. Peritoneal dialysis (PD), on the other hand, could be done at home and could be fitted round my life, and was my obvious preference. There are a number of disadvantages as well as a few advantages of peritoneal dialysis (see Table 5.2).

PD involved having a tenckhoff catheter installed . Although I knew about this, initially I could not bear to look at my body as the catheter protruded from my abdomen. It really affected my body image. I was sure everyone would notice, though in fact this is not the case.

I started using 'manual bags' where I needed to do an exchange four times a day. This is known as CAPD. The bags contained 2000ml and I found that this meant I felt permanently bloated but particularly towards the end of the day. This was slightly helped when they said I could just use 1500ml.

Although I was at home I found the four exchanges a day meant I was permanently clock watching. If I went out I was always anxious about getting back for the next exchange.

I moved to automated peritoneal dialysis (APD), which involved dialysis being carried out overnight while I slept. It was not without its problems. Initially the machine seemed to alarm a lot, possibly because of how I was lying or constipation which is a common side effect of peritoneal dialysis (PD). I persevered because the freedom it gave me during the day made disturbed nights worth it. As I got used to changing my sleeping position and with laxatives and exercise controlling the constipation, the alarms became less frequent.

I still had the bloating feeling as at the end of the treatment I had 1500ml in my peritoneum. However, after some time when the dialysis had been working well, the renal team agreed I could be 'dry' during the day which has been much more comfortable.

CASE STUDY 5.2   GLORIA

 Apart from constipation caused by PD, the treatment caused me to make significant changes to my life. These included the need to change the dressing every time I showered. This meant that I could not really go swimming or wear a swimsuit on holiday because of the appearance.

Treatment for renal disease invariably involves dietary change; currently I am on a low salt and low phosphate diet. I was given a long list of foods to avoid. I went through the lists looking at foods I would normally eat and changed my diet accordingly. I no longer eat certain foods like smoked fish because of salt and nuts and even chocolate because of the phosphate.

The dialysis fluid is delivered monthly. After delivery I have over half a tonne of fluid in the house. This is stored in a spare bedroom, which makes it difficult to accommodate visitors. Without the ability to store the fluid, it would be hard to have APD at home.

I am, however, still able to go on holiday and I am grateful for that but can no longer do touring holidays as we have to stay in one place. Travel insurance can be hard to find and expensive. I tried to visit Canada but the cost for insurance would have covered a holiday in Europe. I am not on the transplant list and have been on APD for over eight years. It is now part of life's routine. When going to bed I set up the machine in the same way some people brush their teeth though it takes considerably longer. I feel well and know that without dialysis I would not be here.

RENAL PALLIATIVE CARE

The fastest expanding group receiving hospital haemodialysis has been the elderly (Murtagh and Murphy 2008). However, for very elderly patients with high comorbidity, dialysis may not offer a survival advantage and some patients choose not to embark on a life of dialysis treatment. Patients with CKD have extensive and unique palliative care needs, often for years before death. High mortality rates along with a substantial burden of physical, psychosocial and spiritual symptoms and an increasing prevalence of decisions to withhold and stop dialysis all highlight the importance of integrating palliative care into the comprehensive management of patients with CKD (Da Silva, 2014). The focus of renal care would then extend to controlling symptoms, communicating prognosis, establishing goals of care and determining end of life care preferences (Holley, 2007).

Caring for patients on a hospital dialysis unit provides nurses with a unique insight and awareness of their patients' overall health and wellbeing. Nurses are in a prime position to identify patients who may be becoming unstable on dialysis or deteriorating despite dialysis treatment. My unpublished master's study (Heatley, 2012), undertaken in an inner-city dialysis centre, explored the renal nurse's perceptions of the role of advanced care planning in patients undergoing hospital haemodialysis. The study found that nurses caring for such patients develop a 'sixth sense' about their patients when they are deteriorating on dialysis treatment:

> You just know when the patients are deteriorating, you can see little changes because you see them so often, you seem to develop this 'sixth sense' about changes in their condition, that's why renal nursing is so different, we really get to know the patients.

> Sandeep, renal nurse

> I have been a renal nurse now for some years, this helps you develop skills, where you develop a sense that things are changing in the patient's condition, it's not something you can put your put your 'finger on' you just know, it's quite complex really.

> Caroline, renal nurse

Symptom burden in patients dying of ESRD is reflected in those patients nearing the end of life (see Table 5.3).

In consideration of the high symptom burden and low survival rate for dialysis patients, including those patients who choose not to have dialysis treatments, the Renal Physicians Association (2010) suggests that it is imperative that renal teams

Table 5.3 Symptoms in patients with ESRD nearing the end of life

Symptoms	Causes
Nausea and vomiting	Build-up of uraemic toxins
Anaemia	Decreased production of ESA hormone
Shortness of breath	Anaemia, pulmonary oedema, acidosis
Purities	Uraemia, iron deficiency
Lack of appetite	Uraemia, depression
Restless legs	Specific cause unknown, common in ESRD
Cramps	Specific cause unknown
Dry mouth	Uraemia, medications
Pain	Pain is common, often multiple pains

incorporate palliative care into the treatment of patients. Nephrologists and renal nursing teams are being encouraged to obtain education and skills in palliative care, and to develop policies and protocols that ensure palliative care is provided to their patients.

Dialysis is life prolonging, not curative. With the progression of kidney disease, palliative care assumes an increasing priority over curative care and eventually focuses on the dying process.

END OF LIFE CARE

Many patients who receive dialysis also suffer from multiple comorbidities (O'Connor et al., 2013). Patients receiving haemodialysis often report feeling less independent and unable to participate in activities they enjoy and have an overall decline in functional status and quality of life (Schmidt and Moss, 2014).

Withdrawal of dialysis treatment is most often motivated by failure to thrive while on dialysis and poor quality of life. It is also demonstrated by an inability or unwillingness to accept and endure the process of dialysis and the burdens it imposes (Kaufman et al., 2007). The withdrawal of dialysis has increased as a cause of death in dialysis-dependent patients (Fassett, 2014). In this sense the palliative phase of care is short-lived as once the patient is withdrawn from dialysis, end of life is imminent. The characteristics of care during this palliative phase for patients focus around withdrawing from dialysis treatment. This is a crucial time from the patient's perspective, and careful monitoring of symptoms such as receiving adequate symptom management (pain, agitation, myoclonus, dyspnoea, nausea and respiratory tract secretions) are important to ensure quality of life. These are the major symptoms in patients with advanced kidney failure at the end of life (see Table 5.3). It is important in the transition from palliative to end of life care to avoid inappropriate prolongation of dying, achieving a sense of control and relieving the burden on loved ones (Holley, 2012).

The decision to stop treatment should be an informed and voluntary choice. With shared decision making, the nephrologist works closely with the patient and their families and the various members of the renal multidisciplinary team regarding stopping dialysis and planning for end of life care. Without lifesaving dialysis treatment, death is likely to occur within days or a few weeks.

While talking about death and dying can be difficult, most patients and their families find it is a relief to have a plan in place for when the end of their life is close. Planning for care and respecting the wishes of the patient make end of life decisions easier (Rak et al., 2016). Renal nurses are in a prime position to begin the process of planning for end of life care given their unique long-term relationships with the dialysis patients they care for (Seymour, 2010; Yee et al., 2011). Supporting the patient and their families as end of life approaches is reported as being a fundamental role of the renal nurse (Yee et al., 2011).

Once dialysis has been stopped the focus of care is on helping patients stay as comfortable as possible during the remaining days or weeks of their lives. Meticulous pain and symptom management are imperative once dialysis treatment is withdrawn. Without dialysis, toxins build up in the blood, causing a condition called ureamia. As the toxins build up, the patient will experience physical and emotional changes. In the final days, the body starts to shut down. In most instances, the shut-down is an orderly series of physical changes:

- Loss of appetite and fluid overload
- Sleeping most of the day
- Disorientation, confusion and failure to recognise familiar faces
- Changes in breathing (normal breathing patterns may become shallow, irregular, fast or extremely slow). There may be periods of breathing that sound like panting
- Exhaling may create a moan-like sound. This is not distress, but the sound of air passing over the vocal cords
- Changed breathing patterns indicate decreased circulation in the internal organs and build-up of waste products. Elevating the head and/or turning onto the side may increase comfort
- Changes in colour and skin temperature

As the body's systems shut down, the patient slips into unconsciousness and the heart stops beating. Studies into end of life care for patients withdrawing from dialysis have suggested that when patients and their families are prepared for the final days of life it provides them with the opportunity for closure and to say good-bye (Davison et al., 2006).

The long-term nature of renal disease and dialysis treatment means that holistic patient-centred support is a huge part of the routine management of renal patients. Assisting patients and their families in making end of life care plans, ensuring good symptom management is provided, and ultimately supporting and respecting their wishes once the decision has been made to withdraw dialysis are essential elements of care provided by the renal team.

CONCLUSION

This chapter has described the pathophysiology of renal disease and the key symptoms associated with acute renal failure and the stages leading up to and including end stage renal failure. In order to illustrate a full picture, the chapter has included both nurses' and patients' perspectives on living with renal disease and the advantages and disadvantages of different forms of treatment. Treatment itself can cause a burden for both the patient and their family as Siva's account makes clear. In the palliative phase of care, the deterioration in the patient's condition requires effective communication and trust in order to avoid some of the distress associated with patients becoming aware that curative attempts to sustain life have been relinquished and quality of life and comfort care have become the aim. The patient and family are likely to be very aware that without lifesaving dialysis treatment, death is likely to occur within days or a few weeks. Towards the end of life, withdrawing from dialysis involves nurses, doctors and others to engage with the patient and prepare them for the final days of life and give them opportunity for closure and to say goodbye. Knowing their wishes and seeking to meet individual needs at all stages from diagnosis to death are key to enabling the patient and family to experience a good death.

REFERENCES

Ashker, V.E., Penprase, B. and Salman, A. (2012) 'Work-related emotional stressors and coping strategies that affect the well-being of nurses working in haemodialysis units.' *Nephrology Nursing Journal*, 39: 231–6.

Bilgic, A., Akgul, A., Sezer, S., Arat, Z., Ozdemir, F.N. and Haberal, M. (2007) 'Nutritional status and depression, sleep disorder, and quality of life in haemodialysis patients.' *Journal of Renal Nutrition*, 17: 381–8.

Blagg, C.R. (2008) 'Home haemodialysis.' *BMJ*, 336 (7634): 3–4.

Cohen, L.M., Moss, A.H., Weisbord, S.D. and Germain, M.J. (2006) 'Renal palliative care.' *Journal of Palliative Medicine*, 9 (4): 977–92.

Cvengros, J.A., Christensen, A.J. and Lawton, W.J. (2005) 'Health locus of control and depression in chronic kidney disease: a dynamic perspective.' *Journal of Health Psychology, 10*: 677–86.

Da Silva, M. (2014) 'Supportive care in advanced kidney disease: patient attitudes and experiences.' *Journal of Renal Care* supplement, *40* (S1): pp 30–35.

Davison, S.N. (2006) 'Cross-sectional validity of a modified Edmonton symptom assessment system in dialysis patients: A simple assessment of symptom burden.' *Kidney International, 69*(9), 621–1625.

Davison, S. (2010) 'Impact of pain and symptom burden on the health-related quality of life of hemodialysis patients'. *Journal of Pain and Symptom Management, 39* (3): 477–85.

Diefendorff, J.M., Grandey, A.A., Erickson, R.J. and Dahling, J.J. (2011) 'Emotional display rules as work unit norms: a multilevel analysis of emotional labour among nurses.' *Journal of Occupational Health Psychology, 16* (2): 170–86.

Fassett, R.G. (2014) 'Current and emerging treatment options for the elderly patient with chronic kidney disease.' *Clinical Interventions in Aging, 9*, 191–9.

Finkelstein, F.O., Wuerth, D. and Finkelstein, S.H. (2009) 'Health related quality of life and the CKD patient: challenges for the nephrology community.' *Kidney International, 76* (9): 946–52.

Hayes, B., Bonner, A. and Douglas, C. (2015) 'Haemodialysis work environment contributors to job satisfaction and stress: a sequential mixed methods study.' *BMC Nursing, 14*: 58.

Heatley, S. (2012) 'Exploring the knowledge and perceptions of renal unit nurses regarding advance care planning (ACP) and their views on the feasibility of its implementation in hospital haemodialysis units.' Unpublished Msc thesis submitted to University of Manchester, 2012.

Holley, J. (2007) 'Palliative care in end-stage renal disease: illness trajectories, communication, and hospice use.' *Advances in Chronic Kidney Disease, 14*, 402–8.

Holley, J.L. (2012) 'Advance care planning in CKD/ESRD: an evolving process.' *Clinical Journal of the American Society of Nephrology, 7*: 1033–8.

Jablonski, A. (2007) 'The multidimensional characteristics of symptoms reported by patients on haemodialysis.' *Nephrology Nursing Journal, 34* (1): 29–37.

Jenkins, K., Bennett, L., Lancaster, L., O'Donoghue, D. and Carillo, F. (2002) 'Improving the nurse–patient relationship: a multi-faceted approach.' *EDTNA ERCA Journal, 28* (3): 145–50.

Kaufman, R., Ann, J., Russa, J.K. and Shim S. (2007) 'The value of "life at any cost": talk about stopping kidney dialysis.' *Social Science and Medicine, 64* (11): 2236–47.

Kutner, N.G., Zhang, R., McClellan, W.M. and Cole, S.A. (2009) 'Psychosocial predictors of non-compliance in haemodialysis and peritoneal dialysis patients.' *Nephrology Dialysis Transplant, 17*: 93–9.

Liyanage, T., Ninomiya, T., Jha, V., Neal, B., Patrice, H.M. and Okpechi, I. (2015) 'Worldwide access to treatment for end-stage kidney disease: a systematic review.' *The Lancet, 385*: 1975–82.

Muringai, T., Noble, H., McGowan, A. and Channey, M. (2008) 'Dialysis access and the impact on body image: role of the nephrology nurse.' *British Journal of Nursing, 17* (6): 362–6.

Murtagh, F.E.M., Addington-Hall, J. and Higginson, I.J. (2006) 'The prevalence of symptoms in end stage renal disease: a systematic review.' *Advances in Chronic Kidney Disease, 14*: 82–99.

Murtagh, F.E. and Murphy, E. (2008) 'Palliative and end of life needs in dialysis patients.' *Seminars in Dialysis, 21* (2): 196.

O'Connor, N.R., Dougherty, M. and Harris, P.S. (2013) 'Survival after dialysis discontinuation and hospice enrolment for ESRD.' *Clinical Journal of the American Society of Nephrology*, 8: 2117–22.

Polaschek, N. (2003) 'Living on dialysis: concerns of clients in a renal setting.' *Journal of Advanced Nursing*, 41: 44–52.

Rak, A., Raina, R., Suh, T.S., Krishnappa, V, et al. (2016) 'Palliative care for patients with end-stage renal disease: approach to treatment that aims to improve quality of life and relieve suffering for patients (and families) with chronic illnesses.' *Clinical Kidney Journal*, 10: 68–73.

Reichsman, F. and Levy, N.B. (1972) 'Adaptation to haemodialysis: a four year study of 25 patients.' *Archives of Internal Medicine*, 138: 859–65.

Renal Physicians Association (2010) *Shared Decision-Making in the Appropriate Initiation of and Withdrawal from Dialysis.* 2nd ed. Rockville, MD: Renal Physicians Association.

Robinson, B., Jagar, K., Kerr, P., Saran, R. and Pisoni, R. (2016) 'Factors affecting outcomes in patients reaching end stage kidney disease worldwide: differences in access to renal replacement therapy, modality, use and haemodialysis practice.' *The Lancet*, 208, 211–306.

Rygh, E., Arild, E., Johsen, E. and Rumpsfield, M. (2012) 'Choosing to live with home dialysis-patients' experiences and potential for telemedicine support: a qualitative study.' *BMC Nephrology*, 13: 13.

Saini, T., Murtagh, F.E., Dupont, P.J., McKinnon, P.M., Hatfield, P. and Saunders, Y. (2006) 'Comparative pilot study of symptoms and quality of life in cancer patients and patients with end stage renal disease.' *Palliative Medicine*, 20 (6): 631–6.

Schmidt, R.J. and Moss, A.H.(2014) 'Dying on dialysis: the case for a dignified withdrawal.' *Clinical Journal American Society*, 9, 174–80.

Seymour, J. (2010) 'Implementing advance care planning: a qualitative study of community nurses' views and experiences.' *BMC Palliative Care*, 9: 4.

Trimmers, L., Thong, M., Dekker, F., Boeschohan, E., et al. (2008) 'Illness perceptions in dialysis patients and their association with quality of life.' *Psychology and Health*, 23 (6): 679–90.

United States Renal Data System (2015) *2015 USRDS Annual Data Report: Epidemiology of Kidney Disease in the United States.* Volume 5, Issue 1, June 2015, pp. 2–7. Bethesda, MD: National Institutes of Health, National Institute of Diabetes and Digestive and Kidney Diseases.

Wilkie, M. (2011) 'Home dialysis – an international perspective'. *NDT Plus*, 4 (Suppl. 3) iii4–6, https://doi.org/10.1093/ndtplus/sfr12

Yee, A., Seow, Y.Y., Tan, S.H., Goh, C., Qu, L. and Lee, G. (2011) 'What do renal health-care professionals in Singapore think of advance care planning for patients with end-stage renal disease?' *Nephrology*, 16 (2): 232–8.

FURTHER READING

Davison, S.N., Jhangri, G.S., Holley, J.L and Moss, A.H. (2006) 'Nephrologists' reported preparedness for end-of-life decision-making.' *Clinical Journal of the American Society of Nephrology*, 1: 1256–62.

Seymour, J. (2010) *Capacity, Care Planning and Advance Care Planning in Life Limiting Illness: A Guide for Health and Social Care.* National End of Life Care Programme.

Vestman, C., Hasselroth, M. and Berglund, M. (2014) 'Freedom and confinement: patients' experiences of life with home haemodialysis.' *Nursing Research and Practice.* doi: 10.1155/2014/252643

Wilkie, M. (2011) 'Home dialysis – an international perspective.' *NDT Plus*, 4 (Suppl. 3): iii4–6.

6

PALLIATIVE CARE FOR PEOPLE WITH ADVANCED DEMENTIA

JACQUELINE CROWTHER

LEARNING OUTCOMES

- Have an awareness of the different types of dementia and common symptoms
- Be able to identify the common nursing problems associated with dementia
- Have an awareness of challenges associated with identifying end of life and the goals of palliative care
- Identify family issues and the importance of advance care planning

INTRODUCTION

As the population ages and more people develop dementia, end of life and palliative care issues will become increasingly important for society as a whole, not only in dementia care (Alzheimer's Society, 2012). One in three people over the age of 65 will die with some form of dementia (Brayne et al., 2006). This chapter describes the pathophysiology of dementia and the common symptoms and nursing challenges this condition raises. Dementia will be discussed initially in its broadest terms considering the most common types and symptoms. In relation to dementia, the American Psychiatric Association of Mental Disorder in 2013 changed its diagnostic criteria in order to maintain parity with changes in clinical practice and as a way of reducing the stigma associated with the term 'dementia', which has been removed from the diagnostic manual. The new term used in the *Diagnostic and*

Statistical Manual (American Psychiatric Association, 2013) refers to dementia as a 'major neurocognitive disorder'. The term dementia now includes Alzheimer's disease, vascular, Lewy body and frontal temporal lobe dementia. However, the term 'dementia' as well as 'major neurocognitive disorder' will continue to be used in this chapter interchangeably largely because work referenced in the literature in many cases pre-dates the change and those more up-to-date references have continued to use the term 'dementia'.

The focus of the chapter is on palliative and end of life care for people with dementia and the need to improve quality of life as death approaches, including the need for advance care planning (ACP). Unlike other life-limiting illnesses, the disease trajectory of dementia is often long, protracted and unpredictable. Prognostication of end of life can be problematic and access to specialist palliative care services, including hospice care, is limited, variable and inequitable resulting in negative experiences at end of life (Middleton-Green et al., 2017; Sampson et al., 2006). Palliative and end of life care, including legal and ethical issues, are addressed and awareness raised of different types of major neurocognitive disorders, common symptoms and common nursing problems associated with major neurocognitive disorders at end of life. The needs of family and lay caregivers, who form an important part of the overall experience of major neurocognitive disorders, are also highlighted. ACP is an important part of end of life care. The need for palliative care practitioners to recognise the individuality of the patient and be aware that not all patients experiencing dementia share the same set of symptoms as people with other life-limiting illnesses is highlighted. It is important for specialist palliative care practitioners to recognise the transferability of existing knowledge, skills and expertise to the care of people with advanced major neurocognitive disorders as end of life approaches. Collaboration, partnership and the sharing of knowledge and skills is crucial to the development of good end of life care for people with these conditions, as well as development of the workforce and the creation of positive experiences and subsequent memories after death for the bereaved and professional staff.

AGEING AND DEMENTIA

The older population is increasing globally with growing numbers of people living longer into older age (Office for National Statistics (ONS), 2016a). This is mostly attributable to advances in science and medicine enabling us to live longer with chronic, age-related and terminal conditions. From a national perspective, the percentage of older people (65 years and over) has grown by 47 per cent since 1974. This increase accounted for almost 18 per cent of the total United Kingdom population in 2014 (ONS, 2016a). The numbers of those reaching the oldest ages are increasing the fastest. In 2008 there were 1.3 million people in the UK aged 85 and over. This figure is expected to rise to 1.8 million by 2018 and to 3.3 million by 2033 (Stephan and Brayne, 2008). These changes to the age structure of the population influence both the prevalence and incidence of age-related conditions such as dementia (Wilcock et al., 1999).

In relation to dementia, in 2014 there were 683,597 people with dementia in the UK with this number predicted to increase to 940,110 by 2021 and to 1,735,087 by 2051, an increase of 38 per cent over the next 15 years (NHS England, 2014). Among those with dementia, at any one time it is estimated that 55 per cent have mild dementia, 32 per cent moderate dementia and 12 per cent have advanced dementia. Advanced dementia increases with age, from 6 per cent for those aged 65 to 69 years to nearly 25 per cent for those aged 95 years and over (NHS England, 2014). As people age they are more likely to experience a range of complex, long-term health conditions including dementia, heart disease, cancer, stroke, frailty, respiratory disease and diabetes (Barnett et al., 2012), increasing the complexities of treatment and management for health and social care professionals. People will be living with dementia but it is more likely other diseases such as heart disease will eventually become the cause of death (Kuhn, 2013; Public Health England, 2016). Other risk factors associated with developing dementia include gender (more females are affected); hereditary factors; diet; obesity; cardiovascular disease; diabetes; and educational levels.

Dementia is a life-limiting condition without any curative treatments to date (van der Steen et al., 2014). A diagnosis of dementia reduces life expectancy and increases one's risk of developing other health-related conditions (van der Steen et al., 2014). Treatment options which may help to slow the disease, process and manage symptoms are licensed and available for use globally and within the UK for specific types of dementia. These were initially introduced for use in the earlier stages of the disease process. However, some of these medications are now used in an attempt to help manage behavioural issues for those in the moderate/advanced stage of the disease process. Withdrawal of these treatments when efficacy is questionable can be an emotive issue due to what appears to be a rapid deterioration in a short space of time. These decisions are made considering a person's best interests, all information available and with the support of families and multidisciplinary team.

It is important to note that dementia is not exclusively a disease of old age. There are increasing numbers of people being diagnosed with young onset dementia (YOD) before the age of 65 years (Alzheimer's Society, 2017). As a result of migration and people from different countries settling in the UK there are also increasing numbers of people from black, Asian and minority ethnic (BAME) groups being diagnosed with dementia (All-Party Parliamentary Group on Dementia, 2013). Also worthy of note is that palliative end of life care practices will be different depending upon cultural and ethnic background.

TYPES OF DEMENTIA

There are many different types of dementia. It is not a single illness and 'dementia' is an umbrella term used to describe a syndrome (Middleton-Green et al., 2017). There are a number of common types of dementia (see Table 6.1) and not everyone living with the same type is affected in the same way.

Table 6.1 Common types/causes of dementia

Most common types	Less common types
Alzheimer's disease (AD)	Parkinson's disease
Vascular dementia (VD)	Korsakoff's
Lewy body dementia (LBD)	Huntington's disease
Fronto-temporal dementia (FTD)	Creutzfeldt-Jakob disease (CJD)
	Posteria cortical atrophy (PCA)
	Learning disability – Down's syndrome

Source: Adapted from Andrews (2015)

COMMON SIGNS AND SYMPTOMS OF DEMENTIA

Alzheimer's disease is generally characterised by its slow, insidious, progressive nature while vascular dementia may present differently on a daily basis and progression is described as 'stepwise'. Deterioration and changes will be observed more suddenly in vascular dementia, usually following a cerebral incident such as a transient ischaemic attack (TIA) infarct or stroke. Following this episode a person will not return to their previous level of functioning.

It is not uncommon for people to have a diagnosis of 'mixed dementia'. This term usually means the person is living with different types of dementia, commonly Alzheimer's disease and vascular dementia together. Signs and symptoms of these two different types are similar; however, presentation and disease progression differ, as highlighted above.

Korsakoff's syndrome is a chronic memory disorder related to vitamin B-1 (thiamine) deficiency. It is generally related to alcohol misuse but can also be caused by other conditions affecting thiamine levels, such as anorexia, starvation, chronic infection and weight loss surgery. Unlike other dementias, if related to alcohol abuse, with treatment for vitamin deficiency and abstinence from alcohol progression can be arrested.

People living with dementia may also experience what is referred to as 'non-cognitive features' also known as 'behavioural and psychological symptoms'. These include mood, appetite and sleep disturbance, increased anxiety, hallucinations, delusions and, for some, altered behaviours. It is important to note that many factors influence and may have positive and negative effects on all behaviours. These include the environment, the way we communicate our needs, and expressions of pain. These kinds of symptoms are not always attributable to dementia alone and are often the expression of a particular need. This is an issue that becomes significant when providing palliative and end of life care, as it is important to know whether the patients' symptoms are illness related or are part of their behavioural pattern. Signs and symptoms of dementia may be similar across different types of the disease. However, they will affect everyone differently, and individual experiences of dementia are dependent upon many factors including age, physical make-up, background and culture, emotional resilience and support available (Alzheimer's Society, 2017). For some it can be helpful to think about dementia in terms of a specific stage – i.e. early/mild, moderate and advanced. This can help with the development and planning of future services and care. For example, it is more likely a person in the early stages of dementia can be included in conversations about future care while their communication skills remain intact and they have the capacity to make choices and verbalise them. A person in the moderate and later stages may, however, experience changes in their communication skills and their fluctuating capacity can result in challenges for carers related to decisions generally. However, it is important to be aware of the uniqueness and individuality of different people, which can cause some patients to experience dementia symptoms differently and at varying points in their disease trajectory. Dementia as a syndrome has a collection of symptoms common to most types:

- Decline in memory functioning
- Difficulties with reasoning, problem solving, language and communication skills
- Altered perception
- Gradual, general loss of skills and mental capacity
- Difficulty maintaining one's independence and ability to carry out activities of daily living independently

Symptoms are caused by structural and chemical changes within the brain as a result of neurodegenerative changes. The cognitive changes arising in dementia are determined to a large extent by the areas of the brain affected by the underlying pathological processes. These processes include tissue destruction, compression, inflammation and biochemical imbalances. As the disease progresses people become more dependent on those around them (Fratiglioni and Qiu, 2013; Nuffield Council on Bioethics, 2009).

DIAGNOSING DEMENTIA

The diagnosis of dementia is not a swift or easy process. It is a clinical diagnosis based on symptom assessment and detailed history. It is often carried out by the multidisciplinary team and involves a process of elimination whereby a detailed physical health history is obtained and other health-related conditions affecting cognitive functioning (vitamin deficiency, depression, altered thyroid functioning, substance misuse/dependence, delirium) are investigated and eliminated. A period of 'watchful waiting' over a period of time may also be undertaken by health professionals in the primary care team. This involves close monitoring for changes in behaviour and cognitive functioning affecting one's ability to carry out daily living activities. Once this period is over and process of elimination of potential causes of symptoms creating concern completed, a referral to memory assessment and treatment services may be indicated. Further investigation by the multidisciplinary team should include more detailed cognitive assessments. These can include brain scans (CT, MRI, PET, SPECT) to eliminate brain tumours as a cause for the symptoms exhibited as well as assessing for evidence of stroke and cerebral vascular disease in order to establish more definitive diagnosis. This process differs between geographical areas in the UK and can be dependent upon local funding and service provision. Due to delays with pathways and diagnosis, service development and changes have been made in some geographical areas. Not all people with a suspected diagnosis of dementia are seen by consultant psychiatrists or specialist services. Advanced nurse practitioners with clinical expertise and skills in dementia can also support multidisciplinary teams in exploring symptoms experienced and give a diagnosis. Also worthy of note is that diagnosis can be delayed due to people being reluctant to explore potential causes of memory problems. This can result in people living with undiagnosed dementia for a number of years. It is also the most feared disease amongst the over 50s in the UK and has recently overtaken cancer, heart disease and stroke as the leading cause of death in England (ONS, 2016b).

DEMENTIA AND PALLIATIVE CARE

The perception of dementia as a life-limiting illness has been associated with greater comfort in those dying with the condition. It has been suggested that acknowledging the need for patients with dementia to be provided with palliative care may, in itself, result in improved patient care as people are then more likely to gain access to specialist palliative care services (Hughes et al., 2007). Despite this, families and people with dementia have historically reported specialist palliative care services being unavailable to them as dementia progresses and end of life approaches (Crowther et al., 2013). Evidence suggests that people with dementia access less care and receive substandard care at end of life in comparison to those who have a diagnosis of cancer (Thompson and Heath, 2013; Hall et al., 2011; Sampson et al., 2006).

When considering definitions of palliative care it is easy to align these with dementia and the goals of person-centred and relationship-centred dementia care (Kitwood, 1997; Nolan et al., 2006) from the point of initial diagnosis. People visit their GP for help with troublesome symptoms (cognitive, memory, behavioural issues) that require a holistic approach to management and palliation, usually long term and for the rest of life. Traditional specialist palliative care services tend to be time limited due to the nature of diagnosis and disease trajectories of other life-limiting conditions. One of the difficulties with applying traditional models of palliative and end of life care to dementia is the unpredictable and lengthy nature of the dementia disease trajectory (Middleton-Green et al., 2017). Palliative care for patients with dementia can be a challenge for clinicians. Assessment of symptoms and response to interventions in patients who may not be able to express their needs is difficult and recognising patients who are entering the terminal phase is complex. This may be complicated further when the person is living with multiple other health conditions, often age related, chronic and long term (Help the Hospices, 2013; Hospice UK, 2015). Those providing services and traditional specialist palliative care services are faced with particular challenges due to lack of confidence in their skills, a sense of helplessness and a need for improved knowledge about dementia and palliative care (Chang et al., 2009). Historically, specialist palliative care services, including hospices, have been renowned for excellent care and support of people with cancer. As with cancer, dementia is a complex life-limiting condition with incidence increasing with age. Nationally, end of life care for people with dementia is on the agenda and has now become a priority (Hockley et al., 2010). It now features in both national and local end of life and dementia strategies (Department of Health, 2008, 2009, 2016). The eventual inclusion of dementia in palliative and end of life care policy and guidance is the result of several contributory factors: increasing numbers of people with dementia; increasing media attention as high-profile celebrities confide their diagnosis and experiences; concerns about inappropriate futile interventions and treatments at end of life; and discrimination based on diagnoses that limit access to palliative and end of life care services (Harrison-Dening et al., 2016).

On a European level, the European Association of Palliative Care (EAPC, 2013) published a consensus statement attempting to define the principles of palliative care for older people with Alzheimer's disease and progressive dementias (van der Steen et al., 2014). This resulted in a model which identified specific goals of palliative care for dementia ranging from minimal cognitive dysfunction (intact) up to advanced illness (see Figure 6.1). The EAPC goals of care include all aspects of the dementia disease trajectory. Focus is on health promotion and prolongation of life initially. As the disease progresses goals may shift to maintenance of function and maximisation of comfort as one approaches end of life.

Figure 6.1 identifies goals of care that include health promotion and wellbeing across the disease trajectory. It is important from a health promotion perspective to include all stages of dementia in the goals of care. The patient's motor skills may remain intact or undamaged and cognitive deficits can be minimal, enabling a higher level of functioning and independence for the person with dementia. The prolongation of life and maintenance of function is a priority when the patient's condition is considered mild and the goal of maximising comfort should become a priority in the moderate to advanced stage of the disease, with bereavement aftercare occurring after death.

In line with the model and goals of care described earlier, the EAPC (2013) identifies 11 domains of palliative care pertaining to this:

1. *Applicability of palliative care*: Dementia can realistically be regarded as a terminal condition. It can also be characterised as a chronic disease or, in connection with particular aspects, as a geriatric problem. However, recognising its eventual terminal nature is the basis for anticipating future problems and an impetus on the provision of adequate palliative care.
2. *Person-centred care, communication and shared decision making*: Perceived problems in caring for a patient with dementia should be viewed from the patient's perspective, applying the concept of person-centred care.

3. *Setting goals and advance planning*: Prioritising of explicit global care goals helps guide care and evaluate its appropriateness.

4. *Continuity of care*: Care should be continuous; there should be no interruption even with transfer.

5. *Prognostication and timely recognition of dying*: Timely discussion of the terminal nature of the disease may enhance families' and patients' feelings of preparedness for the future.

6. *Avoiding overly aggressive, burdensome or futile treatment*: Transfer to the hospital and associated risks and benefits should be considered prudently in relation to care goals and taking into account the stage of dementia.

7. *Optimal treatment of symptoms and providing comfort*: A holistic approach to treatment of symptoms is paramount because symptoms occur frequently and may be interrelated, or expressed differently (e.g. when pain is expressed as agitation).

8. *Psychosocial and spiritual support*: In mild dementia, as also in later stages, patients may be aware of their condition and patients and families may need emotional support.

9. *Family care and involvement*: Families may suffer from caregiver burden, may struggle to combine caring with their other duties and may need social support.

10. *Education of the healthcare team*: The healthcare team in its entirety, including allied health professionals and volunteers, need to have adequate skills in applying a palliative care approach to dementia.

11. *Societal and ethical issues*: Wherever patients reside, patients with dementia should have access to palliative care on the same footing as patients with other diseases which are unresponsive to curative treatment.

Source: van der Steen et al. (2014) *Palliative Medicine*, 28 (3): 197–209

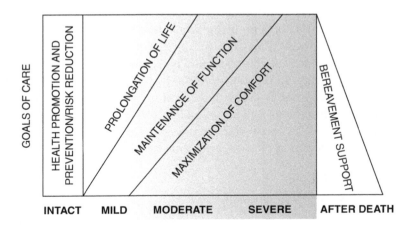

Figure 6.1   Dementia disease progression and suggested prioritising of care goals (van der Steen et al., 2014)

Source: *Palliative Medicine* 2014, Vol. 28(3) 197–209, SAGE Publishing.

When considering the EAPC (2013) domains and recommendations it is important to also consider where along the disease trajectory a person living with dementia may be. Goals may shift and change in accordance with this. As discussed earlier in this chapter, for some it can be helpful to think about dementia in relation to stages: mild, moderate and advanced. The more advanced in their illness the person becomes, the more likelihood there is of them requiring increased levels of support from others including family members. However, a number of people with advanced dementia will reside in 24-hour care. The EAPC (2013) model focuses on disease progression and prioritising of goals. Health promotion and taking care of oneself applies across the domains and goals. This may be more applicable and easier for people living with dementia to attend to independently while skills remain intact and they are in the mild stages of the model where prolongation of life and maintenance of function are the goals.

There are a number of challenges practitioners face with the provision of palliative and end of life care to people with dementia and these include recognising end of life; the unpredictable and lengthy nature of the disease process; capacity and decision-making issues, and pain (Middleton-Green et al., 2017).

RECOGNISING END OF LIFE

The trajectory of dementia is different to other life-limiting illnesses; it can be long and unpredictable (Finucane et al., 2014). Identifying when a person with dementia is reaching the end of life can be challenging and requires the skills of experienced, knowledgeable, competent and confident practitioners. Recognising when a patient is approaching the end of life can be difficult with a whole range of medical conditions and can be a source of anxiety and distress for families. The uncertainty associated with when a patient is dying with dementia can become very distressing, especially when families are informed by professionals that their loved one is approaching death but does not actually die when expected. The person rallies and dwindles for a while longer (Finucane et al., 2014). As dementia progresses, dependence upon others increases and support is required with all aspects of care and activities of daily living. In the advanced phase, limb contracture and stiffness may also be observed, creating issues with discomfort when carrying out personal care interventions resulting in procedural pain. Physical symptoms observed at end of life in advanced dementia can be wide ranging, particularly if multi-morbidity is an issue. A number of common physical symptoms are:

- impaired communication
- reduced appetite leading to anorexia
- incontinence
- pain and discomfort
- behavioural disturbance, agitation and restlessness
- increased drowsiness
- breathlessness

One of the most challenging symptoms occurring towards end of life is delirium (Middleton-Green et al., 2017). Delirium commonly causes problems for people with dementia across the disease trajectory. It can be a major source of anxiety and distress for the person who may experience an exacerbation of symptoms such as hallucinations and delusions and acute altered perceptions of reality. Delirium can create issues within different care environments, and choice of treatment and management needs careful consideration, particularly the use of anti-psychotic medications (Middleton-Green et al., 2017). When occurring as end of life approaches, delirium can be attributable to a number of factors including compromised nutritional and hydration status, and toxicity due to the use of opioids. The presence of delirium complicates symptom assessment and management further at end of life. Guidance developed for the management of delirium (NICE, 2010) does not cover issues specific to end of life care. When a person is considered to be in the palliative phase of their illness, decisions to cease all invasive, corrective treatments (full prescribed medication review) are made and emphasis placed upon symptom management (breathlessness, excessive secretions, agitation) and comfort (Middleton-Green, 2017). When infection, dehydration, malnutrition, anaemia and electrolyte imbalance due to the dying phase are no longer reversible, delirium can cloud and dominate the clinical picture. In such instances, consideration should be given to the use of anti-psychotic medications with a lower threshold in order to alleviate distress unresolved by other means (Treloar et al., 2010).

Prognostic indicators developed in an attempt to support and guide good practice appear to have been more reliable in identifying people with dementia at low risk of dying than those at higher risk of death (Xie et al., 2008). Being aware of the impact of acute illnesses in addition to dementia should alert clinicians to the possibility that a person with dementia may be nearing end of life. Acute physical illness, such as pneumonia, urinary tract infection and recurrent hospital admissions may be an indicator of imminent death in people with advanced dementia (Mitchell et al., 2009; Morrison and Siu, 2000; Sampson et al., 2009). Clinical judgement, information/life history, discussions with families and carers and taking opportunities to reassess or shift the goals of care towards a more palliative approach, especially at times of acute, inter-current illness or care transition may be a more practical, realistic and reliable approach to adopt. There is very little evidence to suggest active, invasive interventions such as artificial hydration and nutrition or hospital admission prolong or improve quality of life in people with dementia. However, there is growing interest in the benefits of a palliative approach for frail older people living with advanced dementia.

PALLIATIVE CARE AT THE END OF LIFE

Person-centred assessment of symptoms and maintenance of dignity and wellbeing is good practice and an integral part of the palliative approach to end of life. Physical symptoms most common and which may be present towards end of life in dementia have been highlighted earlier with one of the most complex ones to assess and treat being physical pain. Pain is often under detected and under treated in dementia; it is important to accurately assess and implement the correct management plan and pain control (Sampson et al., 2006).

PAIN ASSESSMENT

The gold standard for pain assessment is verbal self-report (Puntilo et al., 2017). Some people with dementia, particularly those in the earlier stage, whose communications skills remain intact, may be able to verbally communicate the presence of pain. However, others are unable to and observation of behaviour remains an integral and important part of pain assessment. Altered behaviour such as aggression, irritation, shouting and restlessness can be an indication of pain in people with dementia who are unable to verbally report physical pain. Cognitive ability may fluctuate and although a person can verbally report physical pain on some occasions, on others they are unable to. The presence of pain on occasions may be so overwhelming it affects a person's ability to respond to pain assessment questions (Middleton-Green et al., 2017).

The gold standard verbal self-report assessment of pain is not always possible in dementia. However, it is important to ask questions about a person's experience of pain regardless of how advanced the disease is. Different language and terms than the more familiar ones such as 'aching', 'hurting', 'sore' and 'uncomfortable' may be needed with those whose communication skills may be altered, and the word 'pain' should be reserved for more acute episodes (Middleton-Green et al., 2017). People with dementia who are able to communicate verbally may benefit from supportive communication techniques such as gestures, visual aids and short questions.

There are a number of pain assessment tools available to use with people with dementia. The most frequently used include the Abbey Pain Scale (dementia specific); Pain Assessment in Advanced Dementia (PAINAD) and the Disability Distress Assessment Tool (DisDAT), the latter being developed for those with a learning disability. It is also a more detailed, longer assessment tool, the others being brief. Jordan et al. (2012) identified that the PAINAD also picks up distress and the DisDAT picks up a broader range of signs of pain.

Information obtained from families and those close to the person with dementia are an integral part of the assessment process. This can help guide clinicians in treatment and management decisions.

LIFE HISTORY AND SYMPTOM ASSESSMENT

Life history work for people with dementia and their caregivers, as a means of enhancing care and wellbeing, has been in the literature for a number of years (Kitwood, 1997; Cayton, 2004; Williams and Keady, 2006; Baldwin and Capstick, 2007; Bruce and Schweitzer, 2008). This continues to have relevance at end of life, and information gathered from families and carers who know the person well can support the comprehensive, holistic assessment of the whole person and symptoms experienced as end of life approaches. Information gathered from family carers about how the person expressed a particular need prior to the onset of dementia can be very helpful in supporting care and treatment decisions the person with dementia is no longer able to contribute to. Once a comprehensive, holistic assessment has been undertaken, a referral to local specialist palliative care services should be made for advice with future management of symptoms and end of life phase.

It is important to be aware of the value of non-pharmacological interventions as part of the palliative care plan. Interventions such as Namaste (Simard, 2007) were initially developed as a model of care for those with advanced dementia nearing end of life. Namaste is a model of care that focuses on the senses of those with advanced dementia and is used as a means to reconnect with the person who is non-communicative. It is usually delivered by formal carers but is also an excellent way of engaging families and those close to the person with dementia with them at a difficult time. Although initially developed for people with dementia, Namaste can be applied and used with those experiencing other life-limiting conditions.

THE ROLE OF CARERS IN PALLIATIVE AND END OF LIFE CARE AND DEMENTIA

There are approximately 700,000 family carers of people with dementia in the UK (Alzheimer's Research, 2015). People close to the person with dementia find themselves providing increasing amounts of care and support as the disease progresses, saving the UK economy an estimated £8 billion annually (Middleton-Green et al., 2017). However, this does have other cost implications for the economy as caring over long periods of time, managing difficult situations and choices on behalf of others takes its toll.

The complexities of supporting someone in the family with dementia is also apparent as professionals and different organisations respond to the patient's needs. A number of different people will be involved in providing support to the family of people with dementia (see Case study 6.1). Moreover, families often form the key support structure as caregivers themselves or as supplementary caregivers (Costello, 2017).

Case study 6.1 illustrates the importance of family members in supporting people with dementia and maintaining independence for as long as possible. It also highlights some of the challenges families face when dealing with professionals, the complexities of care and the importance of advance care planning and the effect this can have upon people.

CASE STUDY 6.1   SHEILA

Sheila was an 89-year-old widow with one son and a daughter. She had been an active, smart, articulate, well-travelled and independent lady most of her life. She lived in a farmhouse in a rural area supported by her co-resident son Colin and daughter-in-law Karen. Her daughter Sarah had regular contact and also provided support and care. In the early 1970s Sheila

(Continued)

(Continued)

had spinal surgery for a prolapsed disc which affected her mobility. Unfortunately, this left her with paraplegia that was managed and supported by her family and healthcare professionals. Despite her paraplegia, she managed well, maintaining a high level of functioning and independence with the aids and adaptations to her home. Around the age of 78 her daughter Sarah first noted signs of cognitive decline and memory loss affecting her mother's ability to self-care and manage activities of daily living. She also started showing signs of short-term memory loss and anxiety with feelings of paranoia. Sheila thought people were stealing from her. Obtaining a clear diagnosis was problematic. Her GP was reluctant to investigate her symptoms. Sarah noted a marked decline in the last 18 months of her mother's life – language and communication skills became more impaired, anxiety during the night time was an issue and nutrition and hydration had become a problem.

Despite well-known problems associated with provision and access to health and social care services in rural areas, these were provided and included voluntary services. Sheila also benefited from the Direct Payments scheme, whereby people are allocated money from a social care budget enabling them to select and engage with services they feel more appropriate for their needs. Due to a combination of formal and informal (family) carers, Sheila appeared to enjoy a reasonable quality of life. However, she experienced a decline in her dementia following a hospital admission for intermediate care which caused the family to consider 24-hour care as the family felt her needs were now too great and complex for them to support at home. She was subsequently admitted to a care home. Daughter Sarah felt she knew her mother was in the last year of life but other family members had difficulty coming to terms with some of Sarah's presenting symptoms, such as pain.

Important conversations about the future and advance care planning had been undertaken with Sheila and her family. This was requested by her daughter when Sheila had the capacity to make choices and was able to communicate and document her wishes. Lasting power of attorney for health, welfare and finances were all in place and all her wishes were documented for when end of life approached. Unfortunately, the care home and primary care staff did not appear to recognise that Sheila was approaching the end of her life and were reluctant to initiate an end of life care plan. Confrontations and discussions with Sheila's family about pain assessment and end of life care management ensued. The family became increasingly distressed at witnessing changes in Sheila and the reluctance of care staff to acknowledge the family's level of knowledge and expertise in relation to their mother. The family felt they needed to advocate on behalf of their mother as they knew her well. As a result of the differences and lack of trust about the best way to provide care the family were labelled 'difficult' by the care home. In desperation, the daughter Sarah made a self-referral to the local hospice but was concerned that care home staff may intervene and refuse hospice intervention. Sheila was seen by the hospice medical team and the family were listened to and included in the proposed care decisions. To their relief, it was agreed by the hospice care team that Sheila was approaching the end of her life and the necessary medications to support comfort and minimise distress were put in place.

In view of all the difficulties, the family considered taking Sheila home to die but were advised against this due to the limited services and access to these, as well as Sheila's high level of need. In collaboration with the hospice staff, a new place of care was sought due to concerns about continued care in the current placement. Sheila died peacefully with grade 4 pressure sores with her family present three days after being admitted to her new care environment.

Sheila's case study highlights several important issues for carers: the importance of trust; inclusion of families in care decisions; developing and maintaining carer relationships in order to support best possible care for the person with dementia; difficulties in rural areas; conflicts around knowledge of end of life care; importance of collaboration and advance care planning.

It can be seen from this case study that the family had undertaken all the necessary actions in order to facilitate changes and care as Sheila's condition deteriorated. Their inclusion and role was crucial to the provision of effective end of life care. It also demonstrates the importance of including the person with dementia and their caregivers in order to facilitate care and quality of life for all. It is important to listen and engage with informal and family caregivers and those close to the person living with dementia, especially at the end of life, as it is they who have a more intimate knowledge of the person.

Family involvement is central to the care of people with dementia, especially when it comes to decision making about care and treatment. Their role becomes more relevant as the disease progresses and communication of needs and choices independently becomes problematic, especially if advance care planning is absent and there is no lasting power of attorney in a person with advanced dementia who does not have mental capacity. The value of family caregiver knowledge and expertise must not be underestimated. Family and close friends may become, appropriately, the focus of decision making when attempting to act in the best interests of the patient when their capacity to communicate and make independent choices is lost. It is important to be aware that a significant number of carers are likely to be elderly, experiencing their own health issues and struggling with their caregiver role. It is also not uncommon for an elderly caregiver to be experiencing cognitive impairment and dementia themselves; moreover, the caregiver's physical, psychological, social and spiritual needs require consideration despite the interests of the person with dementia remaining paramount (Hughes, 2006).

SPECIALIST SERVICES

Help the Hospices UK (2013) were responsible for a national call for specialist services, including hospices, to acknowledge dementia as an integral part of their future business. Following this there has been an increase in the numbers of specialist dementia practitioners such as Admiral Nurses, based in hospices and specialist palliative care services. Partnership and collaboration between different organisations are key to improving the end of life care experience for people dying with and from dementia and the carers who support them. Carers frequently experience physical and mental health issues in their own right due to the stressful nature of caring. Professionals and paid carers delivering care must be mindful of the whole family unit and the existing relationships within these which, dementia aside, are often complex. Often, services and resources that may be appropriate for people with dementia, including specialist palliative care services, find it difficult to understand their role within the dementia context affecting access to support.

ADVANCE CARE PLANNING (ACP)

Advance care planning (ACP), also referred to as future care planning, is a process of reflection on and communication about a person's future healthcare wishes (van der Steen et al., 2016). This topic is discussed in several chapters and is often carried out at or near the end of life or once the patient and family are aware of the impending death. It can improve the quality of end of life care, whatever care environment a person is in and is aligned with person-centred and anticipatory models of care (van der Steen et al., 2016). The importance of ACP in dementia cannot be over-emphasised. It is important for the person with dementia as it respects the person's autonomy. Discussions about choices such as preferred place of care and death, lasting power of attorney (LPA), cardiopulmonary resuscitation, decisions to refuse certain treatments, treatment escalation plans, best interests, wills and funeral wishes are all important conversations. For people with dementia, these are best undertaken when they have the capacity to be involved and make their wishes known. Due to the degenerative effects of dementia, there may be difficulties with decision-making capacity and communication. Timing is crucial and choosing the right time to discuss ACP with people with dementia and their families may be challenging given the potential duration of the illness. Different opinions exist about when palliative care and ACP should commence in people with dementia: at the point of diagnosis or later when opportunities may be lost due to altered communication and cognitive skills affecting capacity to make and communicate choices. Van der Steen et al. (2016) suggests that any strategies used to initiate ACP for people living with dementia need to consider the timing and readiness of patients, families and physicians to engage in these types of discussion.

ACP in dementia is important for family members and proxy decision makers alike. In other life-limiting illnesses, if an ACP is available it means people do not have to make decisions in times of crisis, avoiding unnecessary admissions to hospitals at end of life and invasive procedures (Costello, 2017). This also applies to people dying with dementia, and for healthcare providers it means the goals of care are clear and offers greater understanding of the person with dementia and their individual circumstances. End of life care should be considered, where possible, early in the course of dementia when the person has the communication skills and capacity to provide some input into decision making. This is also important for families and those who may have to make decisions after the person with dementia has lost decision-making capacity. Encouraging the important conversations and documenting wishes earlier in the disease trajectory can help decrease the stress associated with making those decisions (Volicer, 2001; Harrison-Denning et al., 2016). It should, however, be acknowledged that not everyone is comfortable with raising the issue of death and dying. In such circumstances individual wishes should be respected and end of life care be based on life history, information gathered from whichever sources are available and what is deemed in a person's best interests.

CONCLUSION

Living and dying with the complexities raised by a diagnosis of dementia can be challenging on many levels for the person themselves, families and professionals. However, just as it is possible to live well with dementia it is also possible to die well with dementia. There are a number of people living with dementia who also have numerous other serious and life-limiting conditions such as cancer, heart failure and diabetes, any of which could become the eventual cause of death, rather than dementia. There is also a group of people living with dementia who will slowly deteriorate and progress to an advanced stage of the disease. Dementia will be the eventual cause of their death, secondary to diseases like pneumonia. Providing effective end of life care to people with dementia is dependent upon skilled, knowledgeable, competent and confident practitioners who are able to support patients and families in times of need. Integral to the provision of good end of life care and a good death is ensuring positive end of life care experiences for all. These can be achieved by the development of partnerships and collaborative ways of working in which sharing of knowledge and skills are embedded in practice. The role of primary care is crucial to palliative and end of life care in dementia. People with dementia requiring a palliative approach or who are nearing end of life can be identified by these professionals with support from families and other organisations. With their support, access to the appropriate assessment and monitoring of symptoms can be achieved with onward referral to specialist services undertaken.

The challenges of providing end of care for this group can often seem greater. This can be attributed to some of the complexities discussed in this chapter such as meeting individual needs when faced with altered communication skills and the capacity to contribute to decisions and choices. Above all it is facilitating an assessment of the individual and not dementia alone. It is important to remember that the memories we create for the families of those people who die with dementia will be taken with them into their future long after the person with dementia has died.

REFERENCES

All-Party Parliamentary Group on Dementia (2013) *Dementia Does Not Discriminate: The Experiences of Black, Asian and Minority Ethnic Communities*. London: All-Party Parliamentary Group on Dementia.

Alzheimer's Research UK (2015) 'Dementia in the Family: The impact on carers.' Available at: www.alzheimersresearchuk.org/wp-content/uploads/2015/12/Dementia-in-the-Family-The-impact-on-carers.pdf, accessed 1 August 2018.

Alzheimer's Society (2012) *My Life Until the End. Dying Well with Dementia*. London. Alzheimer's Society.

Alzheimer's Society (2017) *The Dementia Guide: Living Well after Diagnosis*. Available at www.alzheimers.org.uk/publications-about-dementia/the-dementia-guide, accessed 31 May 2018.

Alzheimer's Society (2017a) *How Dementia Progresses*. Available at www.alzheimers.org.uk/about-dementia/symptoms-and-diagnosis/how-dementia-progresses, accessed 31 May 2018.

American Psychiatric Association (APA) (2013) *Diagnostic and Statistical Manual of Mental Disorders*. 5th ed. DSM-5. Arlington, VA: American Psychiatric Association.

Andrews, J. (2015) *Dementia: The One-Stop Guide. Practical Advice for Families, Professionals and People living with Dementia and Alzheimer's Disease*. London: Profile Books Limited.

Baldwin, C. and Capstick. A. (2007) *Tom Kitwood on Dementia: A reader and critical commentary*. Buckingham: Open University Press.

Barnett, K., Mercer, S., Norbury, M., Watt, G., Wyke, E., Guthrie, B. (2012) 'Epidemiology of multi-morbidity and implications for healthcare, research and medical education. Across sectional study.' *The Lancet, 380*(9836): 37–43.

Brayne, C., Gao, L., Dewey, M. (2006) 'Dementia before death in aging societies: the promise of prevention and the reality.' *PLos Med, 3*: e397.

Bruce, E., Schweitzer, P. (2008) 'Working with Life history', in M. Downs and B. Bowers (eds), *Excellence in Dementia Care. Research and practice*. Buckingham: Open University Press.

Cayton. H. (2004) 'Telling stories: choices and challenges on the journey of dementia.' *Dementia, 3*(1):9–17.

Chang. E., Daly. J., Johnson. A. and Harrison. K. (2009) 'Challenges for professional care of advanced dementia.' *International Journal of Nursing Practice, 15* (1): 41–7.

Costello, J. (2017) 'The role of informal caregivers at the end of life: providing support through advance care planning.' *International Journal of Palliative Nursing, 23* (2): 60–5.

Crowther, J., Wilson, K., Horton. S. and Lloyd-Williams, M. (2013) 'Compassion in health care: lessons from a qualitative study of the end of life care for people with dementia.' *Journal of the Royal Society of Medicine, 106*: 492–7.

Department of Health (2008) *End of Life Care Strategy: Promoting High Quality Care for All Adults at the End of Life*. London: DH.

Department of Health (2009) *Living Well with Dementia: A National Dementia Strategy: Putting People First*. London: DH.

Department of Health (2016) *Prime Minister's Challenge on Dementia 2020: Implementation Plan*. London: DH.

European Association of Palliative Care (EAPC) (2013) *Recommendations on Palliative Care and Treatment of Older People with Alzheimer's Disease and Other Progressive Dementias*. EAPC Dementia White Paper. Vilvoorde, Belgium: EAPC.

Finucane. A., Stevenson. B., Murray. S., Scott. S. (2014) 'Prolonged dwindling characteristics: the illness trajectory of nursing home residents at the end of life'. *BMJ Supportive and Palliative Care, 4*. (Suppl. 10) A1–A110.A10.

Fratiglioni, L. and Qiu, C. (2013) 'Epidemiology of dementia', in T. Dening and A. Thomas (eds), *Oxford Textbook of Old Age Psychiatry*. 2nd ed. Oxford: Oxford University Press.

Hall, S., Kolliakou, A., Petkova, H., Froggatt, K. and Higginson. I.J. (2011) 'Interventions for improving palliative care for older people living in nursing homes.' *Cochrane Database of Systematic Reviews, 16* (3): CD007132.

Harrison-Dening, K., King, M., Jones. L., Vickerstaff. V. and Sampson. E. (2016) 'Advance care planning in dementia: can family carers predict the preferences of people with dementia?' *PLos One, 11* (7): e0159056.

Help the Hospices (2013) *Future Ambitions for Hospice Care: Our Mission and Our Opportunity: The Final Report of the Commission into the Future of Hospice Care*. London: Help the Hospices.

Hockley, J., Watson, J., Oxenham, D. and Murray. S.A. (2010) 'The integrated implementation of two end-of-life care tools in nursing care homes in the UK: an in depth evaluation.' *Palliative Medicine, 24*: 828–38.

Hospice UK (2015) *Hospice Enabled Eementia Care: The First Steps: A Guide to Help Hospices Establish Care for People with Dementia and Their Families.* London: Hospice UK.

Hughes, J.C. (ed.) (2006) *Palliative Care in Severe Dementia.* London: Quay Books.

Hughes, J.C., Jolley, D., Jordan. A. and Sampson. E. (2007) 'Palliative care in dementia: issues and evidence.' *Advances in Psychiatric Treatment, 13* (4): 251–60.

Jordan, A., Regnard, C., O'Brien, J.T. and Hughes. J. (2012) 'Pain and distress in advanced dementia: choosing the right tools for the right job.' *Palliative Medicine, 26* (7): 873–8.

Kitwood, T. (1997) *Dementia Reconsidered: The Person Comes First.* Buckingham: Open University Press.

Kuhn, D. (2013) 'Seeking a better way to die with and from dementia.' *Journal of the American Society on Aging, 37* (3): 70–3.

Middleton-Green, L., Chatterjee, J., Russell, S. and Downs, M. (2017) *End of Life Care for People with Dementia: A Person-Centred Approach.* London: Jessica Kingsley Publishers.

Mitchell, S.L., Teno, J.M., Kiely, D.K., Shaffer, M.L., et al. (2009) 'The clinical course of dementia.' *New England Journal of Medicine, 361* (16): 1529–38.

Morrison, R.S. and Siu, A.L. (2000) 'Survival in end stage dementia following acute illness.' *Journal of the American Medical Association, 284* (1): 47–52.

National Institute for Health and Care Excellence (NICE) (2010) *Delirium: Prevention, Diagnosis and Management.* CG103. London: NICE.

NHS England (2014) 'Dementia.' Available at www.england.nhs.uk/mental-health/dementia, accessed 1 August 2018.

Nolan, M., Davies, S. and Brown. J. (2006) 'Transitions in care homes: towards relationship centred care using the "Senses Framework".' *Quality in Ageing and Older Adults, 7* (3): 5–14.

Nuffield Council on Bioethics (2009) *Dementia: Ethical Issues.* London: Nuffield Council on Bioethics.

ONS (2016a) *UK Perspectives 2016: The Changing UK Population.* Available at www.ons.gov.uk/peoplepopulationandcommunity/populationandmigration/populationesti-mates/articles/ukperspectives2016thechangingukpopulation/2016-05-26, accessed 3 June 2018.

ONS (2016b) *Deaths registered in England and Wales* (Series DR): 2015. Available at www.ons.gov.uk/releases/deathsregisteredinenglandandwalesseriesdr2013, accessed 3 June 2018.

Public Health England (2016) *Dying with Dementia.* London: Public Health England.

Puntilo, K., Gelinas, C. and Changes, G. (2017) 'Next steps in ICU pain research.' *Intensive Care Medicine, 43* (9): 1386–8.

Sampson, E.L., Gould, V., Lee, D. and Blanchard. M.R. (2006) 'Differences in care received by patients with and without dementia who died during acute hospital admission: a retro-spective case note study.' *Age and Ageing, 35*: 187–9.

Sampson, E.L., Candy, B. and Jones, L. (2009) 'Enteral tube feeding for older people with advanced dementia.' *The Cochrane Database of Systematic Reviews, 15* (2): CD007209.

Simard. J. (2007) *The End-of-Life Namaste Care Program for People with Dementia.* Baltimore, MD: Health Professionals Press.

Stephan, B. and Brayne, C. (2008) 'Prevalence and projections of dementia', in M. Downs and S. Bowers (eds) *Excellence in Dementia Care: Research into Practice.* Maidenhead: McGraw-Hill.

Thompson, R. and Heath. H. (2013) *Dementia: Commitment to the Care of People with Dementia in Hospital Settings.* London: Royal College of Nursing.

Treloar, A., Crugel, M., Prasanna, A. and Solomons, L. (2010) 'Ethical dilemmas: should anti-psychotics ever be prescribed for people with dementia?' *The British Journal of Psychiatry, 197* (2): 88–90.

Van der Steen, J.T., Galway, K., Carter, G. and Brazil, K. (2016) 'Initiating advance care planning on end-of-life issues in dementia: ambiguity among UK and Dutch physicians.' *Archives of Gerentology and Geriatrics*, 65: 225–30.

Van der Steen, J.T., Radbruch. L., Hertogh, C.M., de Boer, M.E., et al. (2014) 'White paper defining optimal palliative care in older people with dementia. Adelphi study and recommendations from the European Association for Palliative Care.' *Palliative Medicine*, 28: 197–209.

Volicer, L. (2001) 'Care at the end of life.' *Alzheimer's Care Quarterly*, 2 (3): 59–66.

Wilcock, G., Bucks, R. and Rockwood, K. (1999) *Diagnosis and Management of Dementia: A Manual for Memory Disorders Teams*. Oxford: Oxford University Press.

Williams, S. and Keady, J. (2006) 'The narrative voice of people with dementia'. *Dementia*, 5(2):163–166.

Xie, J., Brayne, C. and Matthews, F.E. (2008) 'Survival times in people with dementia: analysis from population based cohort study with 14 year follow-up.' *BMJ*, 336 (7638): 258–62.

FURTHER READING

Hughes, J. and Baldwin, C. (2006) *Ethical Issues in Dementia Care: Making Difficult Decisions*. London: Jessica Kingsley Publishers.

Hughes, J. and Lloyd-Williams, M. (eds) (2010) *Supportive Care for the Person with Dementia*. Oxford: Oxford University Press.

Pace, V., Treloar, A. and Scott, S. (eds) (2013) *Dementia: From Advanced Disease to Bereavement*. Oxford: Oxford University Press.

Salomon, R. (2014) *Seeing Beyond Dementia: A Handbook for Carers with English as a Second Language*. London: Radcliffe Publishing.

Simard, J. (2013) *The End of Life Namaste Care Program for People with Dementia*. 2nd ed. Baltimore, MD: Health Professions Press.

WEBSITES

Alzheimer's Society: www.alzheimers.org.uk

Dementia UK: www.dementiauk.org

Gold Standards Framework Prognostic Indicator Tools: www.goldstandardsframework.org.uk

NHS England: www.england.nhs.uk

National Institute for Health and Care Excellence: www.nice.org.uk

Social Care Institute for Excellence: www.scie.org.uk

Supportive & Palliative Care Indicators Tools: www.spict.org.uk

UK Dementia Research Institute: www.ukdri.ac.uk

HELPLINE

National Dementia Helpline: 0300 222 1122

PART II

SUPPORT FOR FAMILIES AND CAREGIVERS

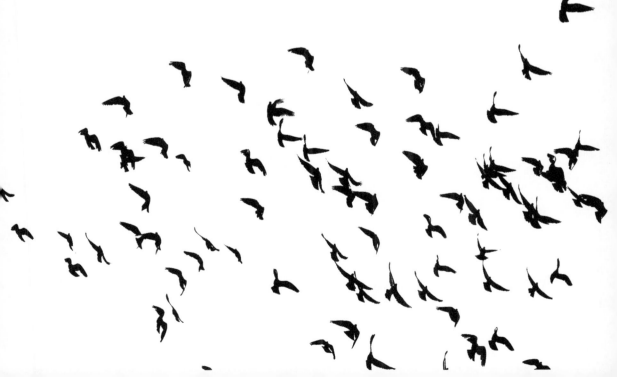

7

SYMPTOM MANAGEMENT: THE MEDICAL PERSPECTIVE

AHAMED ASHIQUE AND JOHN COSTELLO

LEARNING OUTCOMES

- Become aware of how the patients' symptoms are managed from a medical perspective
- Recognise some of the common symptoms and different forms of treatment
- Consider the role of the palliative care physician in providing effective palliative and end of life care for the patient and their family

INTRODUCTION

Palliative medicine is an interdisciplinary specialty focused on improving the quality of life for people with life-limiting medical illness. As a specialty, it is also concerned with supportive care which attempts to prevent and manage the iatrogenic effects of the illness from diagnosis through to end of life care. This requires a careful assessment of the complications of the illness, to improve the patient's quality of life while simultaneously alleviating the caregiver burden.

In the last decade much has changed in palliative care with advances in medical science and progress made in healthcare provision. Palliative care has changed significantly to embrace the challenge of caring for patients with non-cancer conditions and to provide patients with greater choice in where they receive care. Treatment has also undergone change, with evidence-based practice, new care-delivery models and greater continuity between hospital-based palliative care teams, hospices and specialist services. Palliative care has also seen greater involvement and improvement related to families becoming more involved in decision making. The aim of this chapter is to describe the role of the palliative care physician who, as a member of the multidisciplinary team, plays a significant role in patient assessment and symptom management in both the palliative and end of life phase and contributes towards the supportive care given to the family and lay caregivers. This chapter supports many of the other chapters in the book but takes a more medical perspective on the care of the palliative patient.

In order to remain focused on the patient experience, the chapter utilises an authentic case study based on a patient with lung cancer and follows his journey and that of his wife, from diagnosis until death.

BACKGROUND

Throughout the world, palliative care and hospices are highly regarded as providing the gold standard of care for patients with life-limiting illness.

The principles of palliative care include conducting holistic and accurate patient assessment, utilising and respecting the skills of the multiprofessional team and, most of all, focusing on improving quality of life for the patient and providing person-centred support for the family and lay caregivers.

Palliative medicine is a relatively new and emerging speciality, and medical practitioners in this emerging field treat patients with life-limiting illness, not just cancer patients. Doctors in palliative medicine concentrate on symptom management including pain, both physical and psychological. They, along with other members of the team, use effective communication with the patient and family and between themselves, to identify when the patient is experiencing spiritual distress. Together the multidisciplinary team, not always led by the doctor, assist and involve the patient in setting treatment goals. The success of any intervention very much depends on working with the patient and family and developing trust, respect and consideration of the patient's needs.

Two issues stand out in relation to the experience of palliative care. The first is that at some point the patient's need for palliation will change as palliative becomes end of life. The transition experience between palliative and end of life is influenced by the type of understanding and trust developed with the family and patient. Sometimes the discussions about diagnosing dying and planning end of life care are conducted with the family first or, in other cases, if the patient's condition is very poor (as in unconscious), or the patient is unable to express their views (as in advanced dementia), with the family only. The second issue that shapes the experience of palliative care is the choice for place of care and ultimately place of death. Most people prefer to die in their own home, although this is often influenced by pragmatic issues such as the availability of appropriate resources and the ability of the caregiver to manage the patient's end of life care. Most patients die in hospital and some request this as it provides safety and security for them and relieves the family of the burden of care. Increasingly, people who have lived in care homes and nursing homes receive palliative and end of life care in the places they have spent many years, and these settings are receiving more attention in terms of staff education training in palliative care (Nilsen et al., 2018). For a relatively small number of patients, palliative and end of life care take place in a hospice, although for many a hospice provides palliative care and is not the place where they die. Hospices are traditionally seen as the ideal place to die, designed to meet the needs of the dying. Moreover, for many people, hospice is the epitome of palliative care and represents the most acceptable place to receive end of life care. The choice of where to die is a challenging one for patients' families and professional caregivers largely because it often involves facing the fact that the patient is dying.

The principle of respect for the patient's autonomy is paramount for palliative care physicians although in doing this the doctor and the rest of the team may have to rely on the knowledge of the family to guide them through some of the ethical challenges which lie ahead. Fortunately, in many countries palliative care has advanced to the point where the patient's preferred place of care can be accommodated to varying degrees by palliative care services. Hospitals have specialist palliative care teams (discussed in Chapter 11), community services (discussed in Chapter 12) and hospice services providing high standards of end of life care (see Chapter 2). Palliative care physicians work in all settings, although community services providing palliative care in the home often centre around a team involving GPs, specialist nurses (Macmillan nurses) and community nursing services. Palliative care physicians as well as other members of the team provide support, advice, education and training to a wide range of generalist staff in order to share the knowledge and expertise but also to improve the quality of care to patient and family members in whatever setting the patient is being cared for.

ASSESSMENT OF THE PATIENT

An authentic case study 7.1 is used throughout the chapter to illustrate the assessment, treatment and subsequent palliative care of a patient (David), with advanced cancer. David was admitted to hospital with severe back pain, resulting from a tumour in his spine secondary to lung cancer. He was seen in hospital by an oncologist who got to know David and his wife, Sue, throughout his treatment and remained in touch until his death in the hospice 18 months later. The oncologist was aware that the prognosis was poor and David was likely to require palliative care in the not too distant future. He did, however, on reflection feel that it was a good decision to try active treatment. The initial assessment was largely based on listening to David's story. This approach (Carduff et al., 2018) involves asking the patient to explain what had been going on in his life up until the point where he was told that he had cancer that originated in his lung, but had spread to his spine. It was the spinal tumour that was causing him pain. Listening to David's story had numerous benefits, including finding out his perception of events, discovering the impact the cancer had on him and his family, and developing insights into his future, expectations and the understanding he had of his cancer condition.

CASE STUDY 7.1   DAVID

David was a 68 year retired engineer, married to Sue. They had two children and two grand-children. David took early retirement due to back pain which was a result of a skiing accident in 2001. In January 2017, while on holiday in Spain, he experienced severe back pain. This, in itself, was not very unusual for David and he had taken tramadol tablets on holiday which he used to relieve the pain. However, the pain was so bad he was unable to walk to the din-ing room of the hotel they were staying in. On the return flight to Manchester, David's pain increased despite taking extra tramadol. He had to be helped off the plane by paramedics who took him to the nearest hospital. At the A&E he was seen by the medical staff and told he had a recurrence of his old injury and he was discharged with paracetamol, tramadol and an antiemetic. Unfortunately, the pain increased and he went to his local hospital where an MRI scan revealed he had a tumour in his spine. Further investigations revealed that he had a primary tumour of the lung with spinal metastasis; the tumours were malignant. His local hospital prescribed morphine and antiemetics and referred him to the cancer hospital. David experienced ongoing pain in his back radiating down his leg, due to his spinal metastases. He also suffered chest wall pain due to the lung tumour. It was only a matter of days before David received an appointment at the out-patient clinic of the oncology hospital. By this time he was taking morphine sulphate sustained release tablets (MST M/R) 20 mg BD and Ormorph (morphine immediate release liquid) PRN for breakthrough pain. He scored both the pains as 8/10 at their worst and 6/10 after taking Oramorph. The pain got worse on movement. David's other symptoms included nausea, fatigue and constipation. His nausea improved with the use of an antiemetic called metoclopramide. Although morphine was helping to some degree, David's pain was still poorly controlled. There was also an element of breakthrough pain which got worse on movement. As per the WHO pain ladder, David was now on step 3 (WHO, 2018; see Figure 7.3) – i.e. on morphine. In view of his ongoing pain, he required an adjuvant to improve his pain control.

BREAKING BAD NEWS

Effective palliative care involves developing a positive relationship with the patient and the family and maintaining this relationship throughout the patient's illness trajectory. It also includes making an accurate assessment of the patient's psychosocial status and forging a relationship with the patient and their family based on trust and mutual respect. It is also necessary for the patient to feel he can ask questions and seek information at all times (Franklin et al., 2015). The degree of honesty and truth-telling between the patient and the oncology team depends on the quality of the professional team's communication skills, as well as their relationship with the patient and the family. Initially, with David and Sue, the oncology team discussed a plan of care while David was in hospital, although his prognosis was not mentioned at this stage. The team now felt it was important to point out to David and Sue, that his cancer was not curative, although he would be receiving chemotherapy and radiotherapy treatment. It was explained that this would be palliative and its aim was to keep him as pain free and comfortable as possible. Members of the team expressed the view that it was likely that David would be expecting bad news and would not be shocked to be told his condition was terminal, since he had shared with a ward nurse that he felt there was no cure for his cancer. In view of David's poor prognosis, the oncologist sought the advice of the hospital palliative physician, it seemed appropriate that, despite David having treatment, the hospital palliative care team were very likely to become involved with David. After meeting with the palliative care physician it was agreed that the breaking of bad news be carried out with the oncologist and members of the hospital palliative care team. When setting out to disclose bad news to patients, many palliative care professionals find it useful to consider the use of the SPIKES model (see figure 7.1). The issues associated with disclosing sensitive information are discussed in more detail in Chapter 10.

The meeting to discuss David's prognosis took place on the ward. The oncologist introduced the palliative care team members and their role. Together they asked David and Sue about what information he had been given about his future treatment. This led on from the initial assessment where David told his story. They considered his responses and asked him and Sue if they wished to be told what the likely plans were for treatment. David responded positively but said, 'It's not looking good, is it doc!'. The oncologist then told David that despite there being treatment available to ease his pain and reduce the progress of his tumour, there was no real possibility of a cure. This did not seem to shock David and Sue although David then asked, 'How long have I got left?' To this Andrew responded in an ambiguous way saying that it was impossible to say exactly because of not knowing how well David would respond to treatment and how fit he remained. David's wife said that she would provide everything he needed, whatever the cost, and at this point she became very upset. The Macmillan nurse provided comfort, moved closer and gave her a hug. The oncologist said that he could understand how upsetting this was but David said it was what he expected, although the truth hurt.

He also explained that David would be sent a letter informing him when to attend hospital for treatment and that he would come under the care of a consultant oncology specialist. The consultant oncologist also had a clinic at the local hospital closer to David and he would be asked to attend for progress and update appointments. His chemotherapy would begin next week at the chemotherapy suite of the cancer hospital. Thereafter he would attend the oncology hospital for treatment. It was explained that the hospital palliative care team would keep an eye on his progress and that him and Sue were free to contact them at any time for advice and support. Finally, David and Sue were asked if they had any questions or concerns to discuss. They expressed concerns about David getting home and being discharged. The oncologist explained that he would contact his GP and provide him with a summary of David's treatment including his referral to the palliative care team plus a list of the medication that was prescribed. David was told that he would be discharged the next day.

S etting up the interview

P Assess the patient's **perception**

I Obtaining the patient's **invitation**

K Giving **knowledge** and information to the patient

E Addressing the patient's **emotions** with empathic responses

S ummary and **strategy**

Figure 7.1   SPIKES model

Source: Adapted from Bailea et al. (2000)

SYMPTOM MANAGEMENT

Apart from pain experiences, patients with life-limiting conditions like David's experience a wide range of symptoms. The most common of these include pain, fatigue, breathlessness, nausea, vomiting, confusion and delirium (Fainsinger et al., 2017). One of the key roles of the palliative care physician when first meeting the patient and family is to conduct a thorough assessment of the patient's symptoms. This can take place in residential settings such as a hospital or hospice at the patient's bedside, or in an outpatient clinic, or in the patient's home. As Connor (2018) points out, one of the defining features of palliative care is impeccable assessment of symptoms, which include physical and psychological, emotional, spiritual and social symptoms. Holistic assessment is an important part of palliative medicine since there is evidence in cancer patients that poor mental health functioning can diminish the patient's quality of life (Henoch et al., 2011).

PAIN ASSESSMENT

Pain is one of the most common symptoms observed in palliative conditions. The cause of pain can be multifactorial. It can be due to the condition itself and/or from treatment of the condition. Physicians who carry out a pain assessment need to take a pain history.

NOCICEPTIVE PAIN

Nociceptive pain is caused by stimulation of sensory nerve fibres that respond to stimuli approaching or exceeding harmful intensity (nociceptors), and may be classified according to the mode of noxious stimulation. It can also be divided into 'visceral', 'deep somatic' and 'superficial somatic' pain. Visceral structures are highly sensitive to stretch, ischemia and inflammation, but relatively insensitive to other stimuli that normally evoke pain in other structures, such as burning and cutting. Visceral pain is diffuse, difficult to locate and often referred to a distant, usually superficial, structure. It may be accompanied by nausea and vomiting and may be described as sickening, deep, squeezing and dull. Deep somatic pain is initiated by stimulation of nociceptors in ligaments, tendons, bones, blood vessels, fasciae and muscles, and is dull, aching, poorly localised pain. Examples include sprains and broken bones.

NEUROPATHIC PAIN

Neuropathic pain arises from trauma to peripheral nerves or the central nervous system (CNS). Patients like David in the case study describe it as a burning or stabbing sensation. It is not unusual for people with neuropathic pain to have particular areas of numbness in the area of the source of the pain. In David's case it was his lower back towards his left hip. David did not like anyone touching this area even though it felt numb, which is a common response when someone applies even a light touch in the area of pain. The pain experienced by people with shingles is a good example of neuropathic pain.

As well as assessing the type of pain, it is also necessary to assess the characteristics of the pain which include:

Duration – constant, intermittent?

Where does it spread to?

What is the pain score? Use a Visual Analogue Scale (VAS) (see Figure 7.2)

What makes it better and what makes it worse?

Is the patient currently on analgesics? Are they helping with the pain?

KEY PRINCIPLES IN PAIN MANAGEMENT

The control and effective management of physical pain is of paramount importance to patients who experience pain as a result of their illness.

According to Moens et al. (2014) the experience of pain is common in 50 per cent of patients with a life-limiting illness. Moreover, Deandrea et al. (2008) argue

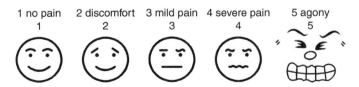

Figure 7.2   Pain assessment –Visual Analogue Scale

that in relation to patients with cancer pain only 50 per cent receive adequate pain control in unselected cancer cohorts. When prescribing analgesia for patients who experience pain, it is important to consider round-the-clock medication. Patients rarely experience pain at set times and it is therefore necessary to pre-scribe pain based on the medical assessment. Round-the-clock medications include use of sustained-release opioids that help with the background pain. Background pain is constant, persistent pain experienced by the patient for more than 12 hours a day. The general principle of prescribing analgesia is to prescribe it with a view to anticipating when the patient may feel periods of discomfort – e.g. if they have told you they get more pain at night, getting out bed or after meals. Analgesia needs to be given before the pain event and when the patient feels a different type of discomfort related to what is referred to as breakthrough pain so as-required (PRN) medication can be prescribed. Breakthrough pain is a transient exacerbation of pain that occurs spontaneously, or as a result of a par-ticular predictable or unpredictable trigger, despite relatively stable and adequately controlled background pain.

Pain relief in palliative care can be complex and may be seen more as an art than a science, despite the technical measurements involved in drug dosages. Ideally, pain relief should aim to provide significant relief from pain without rendering the patient unable to communicate effectively with others. In other words, pain management should strive not to sedate the patient to the extent that his quality of life and therefore his ability to engage with others is affected. Most analgesia has a sedative effect. However, effective pain management needs to ensure that the side effects are kept to an acceptable minimum. It is possible to achieve complete relief from pain without the patient having adverse side effects. On some occasions, pain from certain types of cancer does not respond completely to analgesics, surgery, nerve blocks or cancer-directed therapy. Pain management often involves the use of combination therapy – multiple analge-sics and regular reassessment of the patient's physical condition. It is not unusual for palliative physicians to find themselves changing medication and reassessing the patient's pain in order to achieve effective pain relief by minimis-ing drug side effects without sedating the patient. If the latter occurs, titration of the drugs needs to take place. In a pragmatic way, palliative care clinicians need to accept the concept of 'good enough' pain relief for the patient. Pain relief may be considered good enough when the patient is able to achieve their desired goals without suffering from unacceptable pain and discomfort (Twycross, 1995).

WHO PAIN LADDER

The World Health Organization (WHO) pain ladder (see Figure 7.3) is a well-established and relatively simple approach to initiating pain management. The ladder was introduced in the 1990s and there have been fewer models developed since.

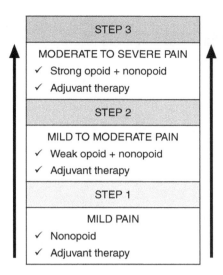

Figure 7.3   WHO Three-step Pain Ladder

Source: Adapted from WHO's Pain Relief Ladder. WHO (2018)

The WHO ladder promotes a three-step guide to providing effective pain relief in adults, with strong opioids, such as morphine at step 3. The WHO stratified three steps in the use of analgesic drugs: Step 1 – using non-opioid analgesics (acetaminophen or non-steroidal anti-inflammatory drugs – NSAIDs), Step 2 – using 'weak' opioids (hydrocodone, codeine or tramadol) and Step 3 – using 'strong' opioids (morphine, hydromorphone, oxycodone, fentanyl or methadone).

However, since the WHO ladder was introduced, there have been few models developed as an alternative to the three-step ladder. Fundamentally, it calls for a multifaceted approach to pain treatment in which opioids are secondary and not primary. They are not to be restricted but rather to be used when necessary. As you can see from the pain ladder, opioids play a crucial role in pain management followed by adjuvant medications or co-analgesics. The most commonly used opioids include morphine, oxycodone, fentanyl and buprenorphine. These opioids are available in various preparations including oral tablets, parenteral preparations, transdermal patches and sublingual tablets.

The most commonly used adjuvants include non-steroidal anti-inflammatory drugs, (NSAIDs). The management of neuropathic pain is better managed through a combination of opioids, and neuropathic agents such as amitriptyline, pregabalin or gabapentin. Adjuvant drugs play a crucial role in the treatment of neuropathic pain that does not always respond to opioids. They also have an opioid sparing effect by reducing the requirement of opioids.

BOX 7.1 MOST COMMONLY USED OPIOIDS

Codeine[1]

Tramadol[1]

Morphine

Oxycodone[2]

Fentanyl transdermal patches[2]

Alfentanyl[2]

Buprenorphine patches

---
[1]Weak opioids [2]Better tolerated in renal impairment

OPIOID TOXICITY

Opioids are a very useful and effective form of analgesia, although increasingly patients are experiencing the effects of their use both short and long term. Box 7.2 illustrates the various side effects and toxicity patterns.

BOX 7.2 SIDE EFFECTS AND TOXICITY OF OPIOIDS

Constipation (onging)

Nausea and vomiting (usually subsides after a few days of opioid therapy)

Visual hallucinations[3]

Myoclonic jerks[3]

Respiratory depression[3]

---
[3]Signs of opioid toxicity. Respiratory depression and a respiratory rate <8breaths/minute can be life threatening. This may require acute reversal with naloxone.

Adjuvants, also referred to as co-analgesics, help to complement the effect of opioids. They help in multifactorial pain, especially if there is a neuropathic component to the pain. Addition of adjuvants helps to provide a more effective pain control and also to help reduce excessive use of opioids (see Box 7.3).

BOX 7.3 COMMONLY USED ADJUVANTS

Steroids or NSAIDS

Tricyclic antidepressants – amitriptyline:[1] dose 25mg–100mg/24hrs

Anticonvulsants[1]

Gabapentin:[1] dose range 300mg–2700mg/24hrs

Pregablin:[1] dose range 100mg–600mg/24hrs

Duloxetine: used in diabetic neuropathy and chemo-induced peripheral neuropathy. Dose range 30mg–90mg/24hrs

[1]Neuropathic agents used for neuropathic pain. Gabapentin and Pregabalin

CASE STUDY 7.1   DAVID (CONTINUED)

PALLIATIVE CARE

David had his first chemotherapy after a consultation with an oncologist who, after his test results, diagnosed him with a stage 4 cancer. The tumour in his lung was estimated at 4 cms. He had metastatic spread. He was given two cycles of chemotherapy and radiotherapy over a period of weeks. His pain subsided and he was able to walk again. However, the pain returned and he was given a third cycle of chemotherapy which eased his symptoms. David was able to live at home for long periods, although he attended the oncology hospital for chemotherapy every week for six weeks, often spending a day in the outpatients department. After the treatment, David was able to return home. He continued to have episodes of pain but he took regular morphine and had tramadol and Panadol for breakthrough pain.

TOTAL PAIN MANAGEMENT

In relation to a holistic approach to palliative treatment it is necessary, as Cecily Saunders (Du Boulay, 2000) pointed out, to consider the whole patient and not just their physical pain and other symptoms. Saunders coined the term 'total pain' when referring to the psychological, spiritual, social and emotional state of the patient. It is well known that the psychological impact of the patient's condition can have an adverse effect on physical pain sensations. Total pain includes the psychosocial effects of the condition which can contribute and sometimes manifest as physical pain. It is hence important to consider these factors when assessing the patient's symptoms and initiating interventions to improve quality of life.

SYMPTOM MANAGEMENT

Breathlessness is a common symptom found in people with lung cancer. It is often due to a combination of reversible causes such as anaemia, infection and a response to chemotherapy, but could also be due to cancer cachexia (severe weight loss).

The aim here is to treat reversible causes like anaemia. Cancer-induced cachexia is difficult to reverse. A short course of steroids may help improve appetite and fatigue. Mild physiotherapy has shown some results in improving fatigue (Pyszora et al., 2017). The goal of the therapy should be focused on setting realistic targets and avoiding unnecessary physical exertion.

Confusion is another symptom encountered in palliative care patients, especially older patients in the end of life phase and when sedatives have been used extensively and the patient is unable to tolerate fluids. Treatable causes of confusion include hypercalcemia, for which bisphosponates such as zoledronic acid can be used. Infection either related to the disease or treatment is another common cause that is easily reversible. Terminal delirium is a well-recognised cause of confusion when patients are approaching end of life. This can be quite distressing to the patients and to their relatives. Antipsychotic medications such as levomepromazine can help reduce these symptoms and thus provide good end of life care.

Using a mechanistic approach to the management of symptoms in the palliative phase of a person's illness focuses on; for example, the causes of nausea and vomiting and the mechanism whereby nausea and vomiting are experienced. For example, haloperidol may be used when the cause is seen as being biochemical such as in renal failure or hypercalcemia. Using this approach, clinicians will use the drug that is most likely to reverse the mechanism and provide effective symptom relief. See Box 7.4 for a range of different drugs used to treat vomiting and nausea.

BOX 7.4   NAUSEA AND VOMITING: MECHANISTIC APPROACH TO MANAGEMENT

Metaclopramide (prokinetic): used in an event of gastric stasis

Buscopan: anitcholinergic antiemetic widely used in bowel obstruction

Ondansetron, granisetron (5HT3 antagonist): used in chemotherapy-induced N&V

Levomepromazine: wide spectrum receptor profile, used as a second line antiemetic when the first agent is ineffective and as an antipsychotic for terminal agitation

Lorazepam: 0.5–1mg for anticipatory nausea often seen in patients who are about to have another cycle of chemotherapy

---

Patients with a range of palliative conditions often experience constipation, which can become a very distressing problem and be caused by a number of other issues such as lack of fluids, poor diet and as a side effect of analgesic drugs such as morphine. Constipation is also made worse by reduced mobility. To ease the discomfort of constipation it is necessary to consider the cause and where possible treat by, for example, increasing fluid intake, modifying the diet or, if drugs are needed, using mild laxatives such as movicol, senna or dulcolax. Another prevalent and distressing symptom experienced by people with cancer and non-cancer conditions is fatigue. This is a complex and ill-defined symptom experienced as both a physical and psychological symptom (see also Chapter 4). The causes of fatigue are multifactorial and can be due to both the condition and the drugs used in treatment (See Box 7.5). Fatigue is a symptom that can and should be responded to as it impacts on the patient's quality of life.

Moreover, it can develop from feelings of extreme tiredness, lethargy and irritability and develop into anxiety, severe frustration and depression (Goodlin, 2005). In the palliative phase of a patient's illness, fatigue can be severely debilitating and impacts on activities of daily living and emotional wellbeing. Telling the patient to rest often does little but add to their frustration at wanting to do more! Treatment includes identifying and dealing with the source and educating the patient to empower them about how to tackle this distressing symptom. Evidence suggests that non-pharmacological interventions such as physiotherapy can make a difference rather than pharmacological treatment with drugs such as amantadine, methylphenidate and modafinil. Gentle physical exercise, keeping an energy diary and a wide range of complementary therapies are reported to be effective (Mücke et al., 2015).

BOX 7.5   COMMON CAUSES OF FATIGUE IN PALLIATIVE PATIENTS

Due to cancer itself

Due to treatment: chemotherapy and/or radiotherapy

Reversible causes such as anaemia, dehydration

Pain

DIAGNOSING DYING

One of the perennial problems of palliative care is the challenging issue of when a patient is no longer responding well to palliative care treatment and their condition is deteriorating to the point where death is likely to occur. This point, often referred to as 'diagnosing dying', is problematic and sensitive for practitioners, patients and families alike. In the past, medical practitioners have looked at prognostic outcomes as a way of determining the patient's likelihood of dying. These include identifying indicators of physical deterioration such as inability to feed themselves or swallow, deteriorating level of consciousness, inability to sit out of bed, and other indicators of physical decline. These are generally useful but fallible. The utility of using this strategy has been demonstrated in many settings such as acute hospitals where it is usual for nurses and doctors to discuss the patient's status in terms of the necessity to carry out CPR if the patient's condition has deteriorated (Costello, 2006).

A more contemporary approach involves asking the surprise question – e.g. *Would you be surprised if this patient died in the next three to six months?*

A negative response indicates a perceived risk of their condition deteriorating to the point of death, in which case it seems appropriate to discuss the situation within the multidisciplinary team and, where appropriate, the patient and/or family. If agreement can be reached then it may be possible to consider a timeframe, such as several months during which time it may be possible to carry out advance care planning. This involves seeking answers to questions such as where the patient wants to be cared for at the end of life and what their feelings are about the type of care and treatment they wish to receive. These things need to be discussed and in practice can be complex and very sensitive. It is often not the palliative care physician who becomes engaged in such discussions although they may be asked to contribute their opinion. Conversely, the patient and family may have previously discussed such issues and have some informal ideas they wish to share with the staff. Advance care planning is discussed in more detail in several chapters, such as Chapter 4.

Once the patient's condition deteriorates to the point where it becomes clear that they have reached the point where end of life care is appropriate there is a need to consider what preferences, if any, the patient has expressed in advance care planning. In David's case, while still in the hospice he had made clear that he would like to be cared for at home. Hospital was not a real option and his wife Sue was very positive that she would be happy to care for him at home as she had a good social network of friends and family able to contribute to David's care.

CASE STUDY 7.1   DAVID (CONTINUED)

THE TRANSITION FROM PALLIATIVE TO END OF LIFE CARE

David's most recent scans showed further disease progression despite chemotherapy. No further treatment options were available to him. David understood that he was entering the end of life phase of his illness. His physical ability had deteriorated in the last month. Previously he was able to mobilise short distances with a stick (performance status 1–2) but now he needed considerable assistance in order to achieve daily activities like dressing and going to the toilet. He was getting increasingly symptomatic. His breathing was getting worse and he complained of pain more often. There were clear indicators of deterioration and it was becoming increasingly obvious that he was approaching end of life. The emphasis in David's case was to optimise symptom control. The hospice palliative care team considered a PRN opioid to help with shortness of breath and pain. This can then be converted to a long acting sustained release preparation based on the PRN requirements. David was commenced on pregabalin 50 mg BD along with the MST 20 mg BD. Over the subsequent days his pregabalin dose was gradually increased to 200 mg BD. David was also commenced on dexamethasone to help with his fatigue. This drug would also have an anti-inflammatory effect which could alleviate his bone pain. David was also feeling breathless. Breathlessness can lead to feelings of air hunger and can further worsen the sensation of panic and anxiety. An anxiolytic drug like lorazepam can help to reduce this feeling of anxiety and panic. David's situation was an opportunity to have honest discussions with him and Sue about his deterioration and the futility of CPR. However, they also needed to be reassured about symptom management that would help to alleviate his symptoms. At this stage, it is useful to have previously discussed ACP in order to discuss and document David's preferred place of care to avoid unnecessary hospital admissions. This should also take into account any other needs that may be required such as equipment at home and extra carers to anticipate further physical decline in his condition. The above discussions should include the patient's family who will also need to be aware of the patient's condition and the likely prognosis. A multidisciplinary approach involving the community palliative care team, occupational therapy, physiotherapy and social worker will help to make the transition from palliative to end of life care more manageable. The above measures did eventually help to reduce David's pain considerably. David was also able to mobilise better. His appetite and fatigue also improved with dexamethasone.

During his hospice stay, David and Sue were given psychological support by the team to help cope with the current situation. They also benefited from the many friends they had who came and visited regularly. David was discharged from the hospice after a few days.

Unfortunately, within two weeks of being at home David's condition deteriorated, mainly due to his level of pain exceeding his prescribed medication. At the same time he began to have breathing difficulties, partly due to the pain and the anxiety it was causing. On advice from the palliative care team at the hospital in liaison with David's GP, he was prescribed morphine with cyclizine to counter the side effects, to be administered by a syringe driver. The community nurses agreed to come and see David twice a day morning and evening to prime the syringe driver and ensure that staff in the community team rotated so that he could get to know all the nurses. During this time informal discussions took place regarding end of life as it became clear that David had reached this stage.

END OF LIFE CARE

This is the final stage of a patient's illness and focuses on David's transfer from the hospice to home where he chose to die.

NICE guidance states that end of life care (EoL) care usually means palliative care within the last few months of life, although for many patients it means the last weeks or days of life (NICE, 2011). Recognisable features of imminent death include further deterioration in performance status in that they are now totally cared for in bed, requiring considerable assistance for all activities.

In order to plan effective end of life care at home it is necessary to establish good links and effective communication between the hospice staff, GP, patient, the community and specialist nurses and family and patient (Ali et al., 2015). Before embarking on end of life care at home, discussions should take place between the staff and family to ensure the appropriate resources and support required. From a medical palliative care perspective it is important to prepare for responses that may be required if the patient's symptoms become difficult to manage and anticipate this by having drugs and other medicaments available. Anticipatory prescribing is often the palliative care physician's responsibility. In hospital they would advise the medical/surgical team or in David's case the GP. The prescribing of anticipatory medication can and does avoid problems such as the patient being in pain and experiencing distress because their symptoms become unmanageable at home (Karlsson and Berggren, 2011).

BOX 7.6   TYPICAL CONTENTS OF A 'JUST IN CASE' BOX

Anticipatory medicines for subcutaneous use (including diluent)

Needles and syringes

Prescribing guidance

Authorisation to administer medication document

Patient and carer information leaflet

Contact details for advice

Clearly, unless requested by the patient and family, the team want to avoid any unnecessary admissions to hospital or hospice. It is therefore important to ensure that there is immediate access to necessary medications (Scottish Government, 2008). In the community setting, resources are available for situations where nurses are not immediately available. These resources are kept in what are called 'just in case' boxes. Box 7.6 lists the contents of a typical 'just in case' box containing medication and medicaments that may be required if the patient's symptoms become unmanageable. These can be kept in the patient's home. The box contains information about what to do in an emergency, which community nurses can discuss with the patient, lay caregivers and/or family members. However, there is much evidence to suggest that problems and emergencies can occur with end of life care at home and access to other drugs required that are not in the 'just in case' box need to be obtained quickly when the need arises by prior arrangement with the local hospital (Wilson et al., 2015). At the same time, access to support and information needs to be obtained quickly as well as help and advice from on-call specialist and community nurses. The BMA in their guidelines for anticipatory prescribing (see Box 7.7) make it clear that just in case medication should not replace the need for appropriate clinical assessment when the patient's clinical condition deteriorates.

BOX 7.7   BRITISH MEDICAL ASSOCIATION'S GUIDANCE FOR BEST PRACTICE

Agree the list of anticipatory medicines locally with key stakeholders

Reduce the risk of prescription errors by agreeing the recommended starting doses and making them readily available to prescribers on pre-printed sheets

Balance the quantity supplied between adequate supply and potential waste

Include equipment and documentation to facilitate the administration of medicines in the 'just in case' box

Be self-assured that the patient and carers understand the rationale for placing medicines in the home

CASE STUDY 7.1   DAVID (CONTINUED)

CARE OF THE DYING PATIENT

As a result of David's palliative care and his illness trajectory where he spent a lot of time at home, many adjustments and adaptions were made at home to facilitate EoL care. He had his bed downstairs and a commode by the bed. Sliding sheets were used for moving and handling (due to excessive weight loss he was managed by his wife, sister-in-law and nurses). Initially at home he was able to sit out of bed, eat and drink with assistance and continued to do passive and active leg exercises. He managed well with his syringe driver with the morphine and cyclizine, managing to enable his pain and other symptoms to be controlled in a good enough way. Over a period of several weeks, however, his condition gradually deteriorated. His fluid and dietary intake reduced considerably. He struggled to take any oral medication (such as lorazepam) but at the same time became more breathless and required oxygen (2 litres) via nasal cannula. He was commenced on 20 mg of morphine and midazolam 5 mg to help with the breathlessness and coexisting anxiety with cyclizine via the syringe driver. David was rapidly approaching the terminal phase. It is important to rationalise medications – i.e. stop those that are unlikely to provide symptom control. The aim of palliative care at this stage was to make sure that medications were rationalised, to stop those unlikely to provide comfort and switch to alternative routes of administration such as the subcutaneous route to provide greater comfort. The aim of care was also focused on ensuring his wife and other caregivers were supported and given consistent information pertaining to David's condition as well as access to specialist services. When a patient is approaching end of life, it is important to emphasise maintaining and improving their quality of life and optimising their symptom management. The imminent death of a patient can give rise to a number of physiological changes such as body extremities becoming mottled, grey or blueish (Twycross and Lichter, 2010). There are also fluctuations in levels of

(Continued)

(Continued)

consciousness. Commonly the patient becomes unarousable, unable to communicate and to swallow medication. Their breathing pattern will alter and an erratic pattern known as Cheyne stoking can occur. At the same time, from a medical perspective it is possible to misdiagnose the symptoms of dying for other problems whose symptoms are similar to those seen in dying patients such as hypercalcaemia, renal failure, opioid toxicity infection, and dehydration (Middleton-Green, 2014). Should there be any doubt, the advice of a specialist practitioner should be sought.

In David's case, as death approached he became agitated and restless, he did not seem comfortable and he began to have jerky muscular movement (myoclonic movement). His breathing was erratic and noisy and his wife and family around him became upset and called the GP. The GP sent the community nurse, agreeing to visit as soon as possible. The nurse who arrived at the house could see the family's distress and the state of the patient and asked the doctor to prescribe sedation.

The GP arrived later and after assessing the patient's condition prescribed a dose of S/C Midazalom 2.5–5mg as required to help control his distress with a 2.5–5mg as required dose of morphine to control his breathing and ensure comfort. He explained to the family what was happening and the likely effects of these drugs on David. After a short time David's symptoms reduced and he became more relaxed and his breathing became more calm and consistent. He passed away later that day without any further distress.

PALLIATIVE SEDATION AND TERMINAL RESTLESSNESS

The prescribing and administration of sedation to a patient at the end of life is a contentious and sensitive issue.

For a number of patients in the terminal stage of their illness, as their bodily responses deteriorate, end of life can produce a number of challenges for effective symptom control. What has become known as palliative sedation is an attempt to ensure patient comfort. In effect, the symptoms that often arise in the terminal phase are pain, breathlessness, nausea and vomiting, agitation and increased upper airway secretions which require management. In the UK, clinicians have reported a continuum that involves the provision of low doses of sedatives to control what is referred to as end stage terminal restlessness or terminal agitation (Rietjens et al., 2018). The symptoms included in this term are experienced by patients during their final days and are characterised by physical, emotional or spiritual distress, agitation or anxiety. Terminal restlessness can have an adverse effect on the patient's comfort and quality of life as well as having a negative impact on the family and professional caregivers (The National End of Life Care Intelligence Network, 2013). Evidence suggests that many nurses involved in administering palliative sedation experienced significant emotional stress due to the lack of clarity between sedating the patient to ensure optimal comfort and control of distress, and euthanasia (Morita et al., 2004).

CONCLUSION

This chapter has given an account of the role of the palliative care physician in the assessment and treatment of a patient with a life-threatening illness. It has outlined a number of supportive care measures as a way of preventing a reduction in the quality of the patient's life and as a way of managing the adverse iatrogenic effects of the patient's condition. The chapter has utilised the authentic case study of a patient, David, and his wife, Sue, as a way of enabling the reader to get a clearer picture of the experience of living and dying with a life-limiting illness. It is hoped that the reader can gain an accurate impression of the role of the physician as a member of the multidisciplinary team who adds their medical expertise to the many contributions made by others to the care and treatment of the patient. Above all, the chapter has considered symptom management throughout the patient's illness trajectory as a way of trying to provide treatment that is at least good enough to manage the patient's symptoms due to the complexity of the patient's illness and the challenges faced by comorbidity. Overall, the chapter has demonstrated that by taking a holistic approach, the patient's illness experience is not just based on physical treatment but considers the psychological, social, spiritual and cultural aspects of the palliative care journey from diagnosis to death.

REFERENCES

Ali, M., Capel, M., Jones, G. and Gazi, T. (2015) 'The importance of identifying preferred place of death'. *BMJ Supportive and Palliative Care*. doi.org/10.1136/bmjspcare-2015-000878, accessed June 2018.

Bailea, W.F., Buckman, R., Lenzia, R., Globera, G., Bealea, E.A. and Kudelkab, A.P. (2000) 'SPIKES – a six-step protocol for delivering bad news: application to the patient with cancer.' *The Oncologist*, 5 (4): 302–11.

Carduff, E., Kendall, M. and Murray, S.A. (2018) 'Living and dying with metastatic bowel cancer: serial in-depth interviews with patients.' *European Journal of Cancer Care*, 27 (1): e12653.

Connor, S.R. (2018) *Hospice and Palliative Care: The Essential Guide*. London: Routledge.

Costello, J. (2006) 'Dying well: nurses' experiences of "good and bad" deaths in hospital.' *Journal of Advanced Nursing*, 54 (5): 1–8.

Deandrea, S., Montanari, M., Moja, L. and Apolone, G. (2008) 'Prevalence of undertreatment in cancer pain: a review of published literature.' *Annals of Oncology*, 19:1985–91.

Du Boulay, S. (2000) *Changing the Face of Death – Pupil Book: The Story of Dame Cecily Saunders*. London: Faith in Action Publishers.

Fainsinger, R., Nekolaichuk, C., Fainsinger, L., Muller, V. et al. (2017) 'What is stable pain control? A prospective longitudinal study to assess the clinical value of a personalized pain goal.' *Palliative Medicine*, 31 (10): 913–20.

Franklin, A., Green, C. and Schofield, N. (2015) 'Compassionate and effective communication: key skills and principles', in C. Farrell (ed.), *Advanced Nursing Practice and Nurse-Led Clinics in Oncology*. London: Routledge.

Goodlin, S.J. (2005) 'Palliative care for end-stage heart failure.' *Current Heart Failure Reports*, 2: 155–60.

Henoch, I., Lovgren, M., Wilde-Larsson, B. and Tishelman, C. (2011) 'Perception of quality of life: comparisons of the views of the patients with lung cancer and their family members.' *Journal of Clinical Nursing*, 21: 585–94.

Karlsson, C. and Berggren, I. (2011) 'Dignified end-of-life care in the patients' own homes.' *Nursing Ethics*, 18 (3): 374–85.

Middleton-Green, L. (2014) 'End-of-life care after the Liverpool Care Pathway.' *British Journal of Community Nursing*, 19 (5): 250–4.

Moens, K. Higginson, I.J. and Harding, R. (2014) 'Are there differences in the prevalence of palliative care-related problems in people living with advanced cancer and eight non-cancer conditions? A systematic review.' *Journal of Pain and Symptom Management*, 48 (4): 660–77.

Morita, T., Miyashita, M., Kimura, R., Adachi, I. and Shima, Y. (2004) 'Emotional burden of nurses in palliative sedation therapy.' *Palliative Medicine*, 18: 550–7.

Mücke, M., Mochamat, Cuhls H., Peuckmann-Post, V., Minton, O. and Radbruch, L. (2015) 'Pharmacological treatments for fatigue associated with palliative care: executive summary of a Cochrane Collaboration systematic review.' *Journal of Cachexia, Sarcopenia and Muscle*, 7 (1): 23–7.

National End of Life Care Intelligence Network (2013) *End of Life Care Profile*. London: Public Health England. Available at www.endoflifecare-intelligence.org.uk/home, accessed 9 December 2017.

National Institute for Health and Care Excellence (NICE) (2011) *End of Life Care for Adults*. QS13. London: NICE. Available at www.nice.org.uk/guidance/qs13/chapter/introduction-and-overview, accessed May 2017.

Nilsen, P., Wallerstedt, B., Behm, L. and Ahlström, G. (2018) 'Towards evidence-based palliative care in nursing homes in Sweden: a qualitative study informed by the organizational readiness to change theory.' *Implementation Science*, 13 (1): 1.

Pyszora, A., Budzyński, J., Wójcik, J., Prokop, A. and Krajnik, M. (2017) 'Physiotherapy programme reduces fatigue in patients with advanced cancer receiving palliative care: randomized controlled trial.' *Supportive Care in Cancer*, 25 (9): 2899–908.

Rietjens, J.A.C., van Delden, J.J.M. and van der Heide, A. (2018) 'Palliative sedation: the end of heated debate?' Editorial. *Palliative Medicine*, March 1–2. doi: 10.1177/0269216318762708

Scottish Government (2008) *Living and Dying Well: A National Action Plan for Palliative and End-of-Life Care in Scotland*. Available at www.gov.scot/Resource/Doc/239823/0066155.pdf, accessed June 2017.

Twycross, R.G. (1995) 'Where there is hope, there is life: a view from the hospice', in J. Keown (ed.), *Euthanasia Examined: Ethical, Clinical and Legal Perspectives*. New York: Cambridge University Press.

Twycross, R. and Lichter, I. (2010) 'The terminal phase', in G. Hanks, N. Cherny, N. Christakis, M. Fallon, S, Kassa and R. Portenoy (eds), *Oxford Textbook of Palliative Medicine*. 4th ed. Oxford: Oxford University Press.

WHO (2018) 'WHO's cancer pain ladder for adults'. Available at: www.who.int/cancer/palliative/painladder/en, accessed 1 August 2018.

Wilson, E., Morbey, H., Brown, J., Payne, S., Seale, C. and Seymour, J. (2015) 'Administering anticipatory medications in end-of-life care: a qualitative study of nursing practice in the community and in nursing homes.' *Palliative Medicine*, 29 (1): 60–70.

FURTHER READING

Ali, M., Capel, M., Jones, G. and Gazi, T. (2015) 'The importance of identifying preferred place of death.' *BMJ Supportive and Palliative Care*. doi: 10.1136/bmjspcare-2015-000878

Costello, J. (2017) 'The role of informal caregivers at the end of life: providing support through advance care planning.' *International Journal of Palliative Nursing*, 23 (2): 60–5.

Ellershaw, J. and Ward, C. (2003) 'Care of the dying patient: the last hours or days of life.' *BMJ*, 326 (7379): n30–4.

Kelley, A. and Morrison, R.S. (2015) 'Palliative care for the seriously ill.' *New England Journal of Medicine*, 373: 747–55.

McCreery, E. and Costello, J. (2013) 'Providing nutritional support for patients with cachexia: challenges at the end of life.' *International Journal of Palliative Nursing*, 19 (1): 32–7.

8

SUPPORTING FAMILIES AND LAY CAREGIVERS ON THE PALLIATIVE CARE JOURNEY

ANNE GOLDEN

LEARNING OUTCOMES

- Develop an understanding of the role of the specialist social worker in palliative care
- Gain an understanding of the nature of social work in the palliative care multidisciplinary team (MDT)
- Understand the role of social workers in supporting grieving patients and family members before and after death

INTRODUCTION

This chapter will consider the role of the specialist palliative care social worker in a palliative care context. It looks at the role that social work plays in providing both emotional and practical support for people with life-limiting conditions and their families and carers, and the nature of some of the support available. It then examines the role of the social worker within the palliative care multidisciplinary team and considers how their role relates to that of other team members. The chapter considers some of the different types of social work involvement with patients and families. Using case studies, the chapter considers ways in which social workers engage with patients and families to offer both practical and/or emotional support from the point at which it becomes clear that they have a life-limiting illness through to end of life and bereavement.

THE ROLE OF THE SOCIAL WORKER IN PALLIATIVE CARE

Palliative care social workers work with people who have a palliative care diagnosis or life-limiting illness – for example, cancer, respiratory disease, heart failure, motor-neurone disease, dementia or HIV/AIDS. They work across boundaries and are often the bridge between health, social care and voluntary and community organisations for clients and colleagues.

The NICE guidelines for improving and supporting palliative care for adults recommend that when people are approaching the end of life, they should be offered timely personalised support for their social, practical and emotional needs, which is appropriate to their preferences and maximises independence and social participation for as long as possible. This should involve a 'holistic' assessment including as a minimum physical, psychological, social, spiritual, cultural and, where appropriate, environmental considerations. This may relate to needs and preferences as well as associated treatment, care and support (NICE, 2011).

Social work contributes to palliative care by making the conceptualisation of death, dying and bereavement more holistic, and social workers in palliative care play an important role in ensuring that the social and family impacts are fully included in services offered (Agnew et al., 2011). They point out that the significance of the social worker's role needs to be made clear in order for them to become more involved from the beginning in the development of palliative and end of life care. Social workers contribute to the important broader perspectives related to the social meaning patient's give to their medical condition and for people involved with the patient. Social workers are also experienced in working with issues of equality and diversity in a framework of anti-oppressive practice (Adams et al., 2009).

Munroe (2005) suggests that there are three forces that shape the role of the social worker in palliative care: the non-medical social goals that the palliative care teams set themselves; the teamwork and skills required to meet these goals; and the expectations of patients, carers, relatives and friends as well as the various palliative care professionals of social work and social workers. Munroe (2005) points out that relieving a patient's physical symptoms reveals the patient's and their family's emotional, spiritual and practical needs. For the social worker, the patient is not just an individual with problems but part of a whole social network, with strengths, resources and attitudes that may impact on the possibilities available.

The starting point for social workers is not defined by their professional role, but rather by the patient and their family. This may start from the time the prognosis is shared with the patient and/or their family and continue after death with bereavement after care (Association of Palliative Care Social Workers (APCSW, 2016).

Caregivers may be defined as people who may or may not be family members and are lay people in a close supportive role (NICE, 2004). It is important to be mindful that people who are the most significant to the patient may not necessarily be biological family members, and that increasingly complex family structures and social networks should be respected. For example, a patient in a same sex relationship may not have the support of their biological family who may not accept the relationship. For some people – for example, those living in hostels or residential accommodation – the caregivers may be their support worker. The focus of social work involvement is to continue to see people living within whole families and communities rather than as an individual with a set of specific problems to solve. This critically includes awareness of a person's cultural and individual identity (APCSW, 2016).

Social workers seek to understand the experience and connections between patients, families and the wider social context of their lives. Support can be psychological as well as emotional and practical, exploring and facilitating change to enable the patient and family to continue to live and die with a sense of control and purpose. For example, supporting discussion around people's hopes and fears and providing information, guidance and signposting around practical issues such as benefits, access to care and possible sources of funding and assistance in understanding and negotiating the complexities of the social care system.

THE NATURE OF PALLIATIVE CARE SOCIAL WORK

While the focus of specialist palliative care social workers is people with life-limiting illnesses and conditions, the nature of social work in palliative care can also involve them in child protection, families and children, disability and other work with adults (Beresford et al., 2008). Specialist palliative care social workers may be involved with any social issues associated with the wider community such as housing, homelessness, employment, substance misuse, immigration and asylum seekers that are encountered by social workers in non-specialist palliative care roles.

Palliative care social workers are registered social workers that work predominantly or exclusively with people living with a life-limiting medical condition. Social work is core to palliative care. With the other members of the multidisciplinary professional team surrounding the person and those important to them, the social worker ensures that services and interventions take account of the whole person as well as their family, however this is defined by the individual.

The regulation of social workers in the UK is devolved, meaning that in order to practise social workers have to be registered with the relevant care council (for example, the Health and Care Professions Council in England) and abide by their standards of conduct, performance and ethics as well as standards of proficiency and continuing professional development. There are also specialist interest associations which support palliative care social workers and develop practice. These include the Association of Palliative Care Social Workers (APCSW) and the Palliative Care for People with Learning Difficulties Network (PCPLD). These organisations raise awareness of the palliative care needs of people with learning difficulties as well as sharing and promoting best practice, to enhance collaboration between all service providers, carers and people with a learning disability. Social workers need to work in partnership with the people they offer support to as well as with other professions, agencies, organisations and the wider community (APCSW, 2016). The setting for palliative care social work can be diverse and challenging. Social workers may be employed by the NHS, by adults' and children's services, by independent hospices and disease-specific charities, and can be funded with money drawn from several different sources.

Specialist palliative care social workers can work in a wide variety of settings including the community – for example, as part of a Macmillan community team or in hospices as well as in hospitals (Hughes et al., 2014).

However, social workers may encounter clients with palliative care needs or those experiencing death and dying, either directly or indirectly.

MULTIDISCIPLINARY TEAM WORKING

Multidisciplinary teams (MDTs) provide a wide range of support to people with life-limiting illness, including practical support with professionals such as occupational therapists, physiotherapists and other health professionals employed by health services, in addition to social care services (NICE, 2017).

MDTs, made up of professionals with different areas of expertise and key skills, are an essential part of providing holistic care (see Figure 8.1). There can often be different priorities and perspectives and often an overlap of roles. This can also be challenged by the person or family the team is working with, changing their own priorities and wishes. Conflicting desires in people struggling between wanting to know only good news and wanting to know as much as possible can cause difficulties for the patient and the MDT trying to communicate accurate information (Cagle and Kovacs, 2009). Cagle and Kovacs suggest that patients and families often need the opportunity to discuss how much and what type of information should be exchanged, where, when, how and with whom. Good communication is therefore essential as a breakdown of communication within the MDT can have a significant negative impact on patients (Beresford et al., 2007). The dying individual and those close to them will have different needs at different times and may require different types of support and often have conflicting agendas (Hughes et al., 2014). At the same time, the role of the social worker can often involve them in representing the evolving needs and wishes of the individual within the MDT (Adams et al., 2009).

Interdisciplinary teams bring different knowledge, opinions and perspectives to the provision of holistic care and the presence of a social worker should ensure that psychosocial care is at the core of that provision. There is often role overlap. It is an important role of the social worker to have an awareness of these issues in order to maintain where the focus needs to be placed – for example, medical care and timely discharge planning (Reith and Payne, 2009). The professional perspective of social workers has much to offer and this contribution should be made in a spirit of collaboration and confidence (Hughes et al., 2014). Social workers can contribute to supporting the MDT – for example, through the facilitation of Schwartz rounds. These are a structured forum where all staff come together regularly to discuss the emotional and social aspects of working in healthcare. These rounds can be facilitated by social workers calling the team together to discuss complex and sensitive case situations where a more in depth focus can be made on clinical and social care matters. For further information see www.pointofcarefoundation.org.uk.

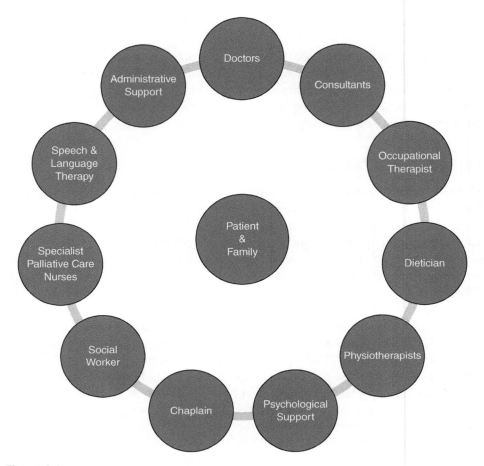

Figure 8.1

A typical hospital or hospice palliative care team (discussed in more detail in Chapter 11) will consist of hospital staff who work full or part time and will include:

- Medical consultant
- Specialist palliative care nurses (e.g. Macmillan nurses)
- Dietician
- Speech and language therapist
- Social worker
- Physiotherapist
- Occupational therapist
- Admin support worker
- Members of the spiritual care team (chaplain)
- Psychological support nurse specialist/clinical psychologist

In some settings – for example, hospices – the service provided by the MDT is critically supported by a large number of experienced volunteers. The approach to practice adopted by specialist palliative care social workers has generally been seen as one based on principles of partnership, involvement, empowerment, respect and equality, where practice was co-produced. This is an approach to social work that service users seem to value and is consistent with current and traditional social work values (Beresford et al., 2008). This includes remaining mindful of people's unique individual, social and cultural identities and contributing this understanding to the wider team.

The combination of skills offered by specialist palliative care social workers makes a unique contribution to the psychological and social aspects of the multidisciplinary professional team (APCSW, 2016). Relationship-based approaches and the concept of reflective practice are established within social work. Social workers are experienced in working in partnership with vulnerable people, communities and agencies and communicating about difficult and emotionally painful subjects and can therefore make a significant contribution to palliative care (Scanlan, 2016).

CASE STUDY 8.1   ADRIAN

Anne had been Adrian's partner and carer for many years. Adrian was in his late 60s. He had COPD and was recently diagnosed with a recurrence of prostate cancer. The cancer had metastasised and spread to his bowels and throat. He had been in remission for eight years and had a sudden deterioration in his condition which necessitated admission to the hospice for symptom control. He was having difficulty in swallowing and digesting food and was experiencing pain in his throat and stomach. He had recently had a PEG (percutaneous endoscopic gastrostomy) inserted which enabled him to be fed via the tube directly into his stomach because of his swallowing and bowel problems. Adrian was a very private man and was reluctant to accept an increased care package to support him on his discharge home. Anne was supportive of this as she also found the visits of carers intrusive. However, Simon, the hospice social worker had discussed the potential difficulties that Adrian and Anne might experience – for example, Anne becoming increasingly tired and becoming unwell or having difficulty or injuring herself trying to help Adrian using the commode, despite the necessary equipment being in place. Adrian gave permission to begin the process of applying for care and to ensure that he and Anne knew how to access the care package when they felt ready to accept it. Adrian accepted regular input from district nurses funded through continuing healthcare, in order to manage his PEG tube, and his indwelling urinary catheter. They also monitored his pain control and pressure areas. During this admission Simon talked with Adrian about his wishes for his future care and his concerns for Anne. Adrian was clear that he was keen to return home but was willing

(Continued)

(Continued)

to return to the hospice for further symptom management if required. He also said that he would like to return to the hospice to die if this was possible. Simon talked with Adrian about what else he might wish to plan and supported him in arranging a visit from a solicitor to rewrite his will. The hospice admission actually helped Adrian and Anne plan end of life care. Adrian was discharged home once his symptoms were well controlled.

After being at home for five days, Adrian's condition deteriorated, and he had an emergency admission to hospital from where he returned to the hospice. Adrian remained fiercely independent, and following a discussion about his prognosis, he decided that he wished his PEG feeding to be discontinued. This would mean that he would no longer be receiving nutrition or adequate fluids and that his death would be hastened. Adrian also made it clear that before the feed was discontinued he wished to marry Anne, which came as a huge but welcome surprise to her. A wedding was arranged at the hospice as Adrian was unable to move from his bed to travel to a registry office. Both Simon and the hospice chaplain, along with the nurses, supported Anne and Adrian with planning the ceremony, which was both a joyful and sad experience with moments of great shared humour. Anne was also able to make good use of the support offered to her in managing very conflicting emotions during this time of both great happiness alongside the sadness of anticipating Adrian's imminent death.

The situation was complicated by the disapproval of the wedding from some members of Adrian's family, which was clearly voiced, and they also questioned whether he was well enough to make the decision to marry. There was therefore a need for clarity around Adrian's wishes regarding his will, as getting married would negate his recently made will. As Adrian was barely able to speak at this point it was necessary to ensure that his mental capacity was carefully documented to guard against any future challenges to either the validity of the marriage or his new will. Balancing these practical considerations alongside planning the very special and personal ceremony felt challenging due to Adrian's deteriorating levels of energy and Simon's reluctance to intrude on their time together. Due to the relationship and trust that Simon had built up with Anne and Adrian over both admissions, Anne and Adrian were appreciative of the need for difficult conversations and of the support offered. The wedding was a very moving and memorable day. Adrian's feed was stopped in accordance with his wishes and he died four days later. Both Simon and the hospice chaplain were able to offer Anne ongoing support after Adrian's death.

REFLECTIONS ON ADRIAN'S EXPERIENCE

Reflecting on Adrian's situation, two key issues stand out. First, Adrian was in receipt of continuing healthcare funding, which enabled his complex care needs to be met at home. Second, the issue of his mental capacity was raised by his family in relation to his marriage and his will. NHS continuing healthcare funding is available to adults over the age of 18 who have a primary healthcare need due to disability or illness.

BOX 8.1   ASSESSMENT CRITERIA FOR NHS CONTINUING HEALTHCARE

- Behaviour
- Cognition (understanding)
- Communication*
- Psychological/emotional needs
- Mobility*
- Nutrition*
- Continence*
- Skin integrity (including wounds and ulcers)*
- Breathing
- Symptom control*
- Altered state of consciousness
- Other significant need

*These items applied to Adrian

NHS continuing healthcare (NHS CHC) is a package of care for adults aged 18 or over which is arranged and funded solely by the NHS. In order to receive NHS CHC funding individuals have to be assessed by clinical commissioning groups (CCGs) according to a legally prescribed decision-making process to determine whether the individual has a primary health need. The nature, intensity, complexity and unpredictability of the individual's needs are taken into consideration. The funding is not means tested. All eligible people must first be assessed as to the level and nature of their care needs. If these are primarily social care needs involving activities of daily living (personal care such as washing, dressing and meals) support may be accessed via the local authority or privately. If the primary care need is medical and meets the necessary criteria (see Box 8.1) the care may be funded by the CCG where the individual is resident. The funding may be received for care at home or in a nursing home if required. In Adrian's case, Simon facilitated the assessment while he was at the hospice. The areas of need are assessed and applicants for continuing healthcare funding have to meet threshold criteria. In Adrian's case, because he was nearing the end of life it was possible to make a fast track application to facilitate a timely response.

Adrian was able to meet the criteria in all these processes. Simon had to ensure that Adrian and Anne understood the application process. Because Adrian was unable to speak clearly, care had to be taken to ensure that he was able to fully express his views. Due to the possibility of his capacity being questioned it was important that this was fully documented. It is also necessary that consent is established when a patient is moved from one place of care to another. If a person is not able to consent to the move, a best interest decision should be made, unless there is a power of attorney for health and welfare in place (see Chapter 6), and a Deprivation of Liberty order applied for. It is frequently the role of the social worker to support the family through this complicated process at a time when they are experiencing great emotional stress and uncertainty. Box 8.2 outlines the five principles involved in mental capacity assessment. The purpose is to protect individuals who lack capacity.

BOX 8.2   PRINCIPLES OF THE MENTAL CAPACITY ACT 2005 (ENGLAND AND WALES)

The following principles apply for the purposes of this Act.

1.   A person must be assumed to have capacity unless it is established that he lacks capacity.
2.   A person is not to be treated as unable to make a decision unless all practicable steps to help him to do so have been taken without success.
3.   A person is not to be treated as unable to make a decision merely because he makes an unwise decision.
4.   An act done, or decision made, under this Act for or on behalf of a person who lacks capacity must be done, or made, in the person's best interests.
5.   Before the act is done, or the decision is made, regard must be had to whether the purpose for which it is needed can be as effectively achieved in a way that is less restrictive of the person's rights and freedom of action.

Reproduced with permission under the under the Open Government Licence v3.0.

Capacity is decision specific – that is, it refers to the particular decision being made at a particular time and a person must be assumed to have capacity unless there is reason to believe otherwise. This involves the 'two stage test'. First, is there an impairment of or disturbance in the functioning of a person's mind or brain due to illness or disability which may or may not be permanent? If this is the case, it must be considered whether the impairment or disturbance is sufficient that the person lacks the capacity to make a particular decision. If an individual is deemed to lack capacity it is necessary to prove and record that the individual is unable to understand the relevant information, retain that information, use or weigh it in making a decision, or is unable to communicate his decision by any means.

Any wishes previously expressed by the person prior to losing capacity must be taken into account, as must any views that may be held by those involved with the person. However, it is only the advance decision to refuse treatment and the decision of a lasting power of attorney (LPA) that is legally binding.

The person assessing capacity can be the person most relevant to the decision to be made – for example, a doctor or nurse for medical treatment or a social worker regarding consent to an application for funding or future place of care. If a person is found not to have capacity a best interest decision should be made in line with the above principles of the MCA. Case study 8.2 illustrates some of the principles involved in mental capacity assessment.

CASE STUDY 8.2   MARJORIE

Marjorie was a very independent woman who had lived alone for many years. She managed her degenerative heart condition and was on constant oxygen and no longer able to move from her chair without assistance. She slept in her chair as this was the most comfortable position. The area of the city where she lived had no care agency that would undertake visits after 8.00 p.m., so Marjorie was left alone overnight until 7.00 the following morning. Due to her chronic breathlessness, communication was a huge effort for her and words were precious. She was unable to use the phone or a call alarm to summon help, or to take medication without assistance. As her condition deteriorated she reluctantly agreed to be admitted to the hospice for symptom control.

The MDT were extremely concerned at the prospect of Marjorie dying in distress at home, alone and with no access to any end of life medication to relieve her symptoms. However, her wishes were clear and the team were committed to finding the best way to support her. In order to ensure that she fully understood the probable outcome of her decision, dying alone at home with no symptom-relieving medication, it was important to ensure that she was fully aware of the situation she would be in, the limitations of the support she would receive at home and the likely manner of her death. In order to have these conversations in a way that was supportive and sensitive to her situation as well as being honest but not causing her unnecessary distress, the discussions with Marjorie were held on a one-to-one basis with her, allowing her to take the lead and take things at her own pace. She remained clear that her wish was to return home, and she realised that the 'window of opportunity' (the time she had left where this would be possible) was short. She was clear what the MDT were trying to do to support her and that she did not want the team to worry about her unduly. She was also tolerant of the difficulties in negotiating the care system. The CCG who were funding the CHC package to enable Marjorie to return home were very concerned to ensure that she had the capacity to make this decision and the social worker was able to support her in communicating her wishes clearly. Although her decision was the cause of some concern and may have been regarded by some as unwise, her wishes were supported. Marjorie was discharged home and found by the carers one morning having died, as she wished, at home.

PRACTICAL ISSUES IN PALLIATIVE CARE SOCIAL WORK

When care and treatment are palliative, social work with the family can involve consideration of many practical issues. Communication skills and difficult conversations are a routine part of social work practice. Many people are unaware of their rights under the Mental Capacity Act 2005 to make plans in advance and may not be involved in discussions about their wishes (Chaddock, 2016; HM Government, 2005). Although advanced care planning is not exclusively a social work role, the skills and expertise that social workers can bring to this mean that they have much to contribute (APCSW, 2016). Social workers may also provide support and guidance around the things that need to be put in place for children if, for example, a single parent has not considered who will look after their child after they die.

For example, in some cases, a palliative care diagnosis can alter the social role of the patient. When a patient who has been the sole wage earner loses their income, they may become increasingly reliant on practical support from their partner. The assumption might be made that the husband or wife is perceived to be his carer rather than their partner. This change in roles can complicate decisions around care and increase both the patient's and family's distress. Individual relationships vary greatly and it should not be assumed that it is appropriate for partners to provide care, particularly of a personal nature. Working systemically with patients and families can make a vital contribution to both the patient and the family. One area in which social workers can provide much needed practical support is assessment of benefit eligibility.

BENEFITS

The role of the palliative care social worker can have significant effects in relation to supporting an individual's personal capacity, reducing social isolation, increasing support for carers, reducing anxieties around practical concerns and providing support with medical issues (Beresford et al., 2007). The evidence suggests that while dying, death and bereavement tend to be seen as primarily emotional issues, the financial and practical issues that arise can be considerable.

However, the UK benefits system is complex and can be hard to negotiate, particularly at a time when people are struggling to deal with physical and emotional distress. There are various benefits that people with life-limiting conditions may be entitled to. At time of writing these include personal independence payments (PIPs) for people needing support with care. People over the age of 65 may be entitled to attendance allowance if they need help with personal care. If people have a time-limited prognosis of less than six months, a specialist nurse or a doctor can complete what is called a special rules application, or DSS 1500, which fast-tracks the application process, enabling much-needed funding to become available more quickly.

FINANCIAL AND EMPLOYMENT SUPPORT

Living with a life-limiting illness can cause considerable anxiety and distress irrespective of the condition. The physical, emotional and financial cost of caring can be considerable when the patient has a neurological disease such as motor neurone disease, and for many years be unable to work and increasingly need more social support (Smith et al., 2012). It is difficult to provide quantitative data on human suffering and the economic cost of living with a terminal illness or caring for someone with a life-limiting illness. Some of the major financial implications of living with a palliative diagnosis are typically housing adaptations and adapting or buying a vehicle. Regular costs include care costs and paying for extra assistance around the home (e.g. with laundry, gardening). Enhanced costs are those that increase as a result of having the disease, the biggest typically being energy bills and travel insurance (Reith and Payne, 2009).

People also struggle to pay bills, which can increase due to being at home more, feeling the cold and possibly increased laundry bills. It may be necessary to buy replacement clothing due to weight loss or a change in body shape, for example due to lymphodema or steroid treatment (which can cause weight gain). Food bills may increase due to restricted ability to get to the shops or not wishing to cook. Symptoms such as fatigue or having other caring responsibilities often cause a lack of motivation. Other physical issues such as changes in taste (e.g. due to chemotherapy) or the ability to swallow foods of certain consistencies can result in buying more expensive processed food. Social workers can support people in addressing these difficulties through, for example, benefits applications and letters requesting financial help to charities and in some situations referrals to food banks.

Issues around employment rights and pensions can also cause difficulty and uncertainty for people with a life-limiting illness. Social workers are able to offer support and signpost people to specialist support. Grants and other forms of financial support may also be available. As well as practical support, they can advise on personal and domestic care – for example, relating to caregivers and patients who wish to maintain independent living, including home adaptations and the provision of equipment. Social workers have extensive experience in access to welfare and benefit services and advising on how to protect the rights of vulnerable adults or children of a family member approaching the end of life. Social workers in palliative care are also able to offer a range of supportive services, both practical and emotional, to caregivers of adults and children approaching end of life. Amongst the services they can advise upon are respite and day care/therapy in social and healthcare settings and care home placements (Adams et al., 2009).

SOCIAL WORK FACILITATION OF HOSPITAL DISCHARGE

Social workers are often at the edge of organisational requirements to achieve a timely discharge from the organisation's perspective. There is always a waiting list of people in very difficult circumstances urgently requiring admission and there is a need to justify length of stay to the CCG. This can be a difficult negotiation when trying to support the needs of the patients, carers and families. Patients can also struggle hugely with the financial implications of moving from a hospice to a nursing home or home. Constant changes in the thresholds for receiving care and funding, from both local authorities and health, can lead to a high level of anxiety, often around the financial implications for the rest of the family after the person has died, for example if the inheritance is spent on care or the family home has to be sold.

If people are financially assessed as being able to partially or fully fund their own care this can cause considerable emotional impact. The need for sole owner occupiers to sell the family home to fund nursing home care at a time when they are experiencing a huge sense of loss of control and identity can have a very negative emotional effect. This may also impact significantly both emotionally and financially on the children, who may be losing their family home and the inheritance that the person had planned to leave. The author has experienced situations where people have refused care due to the financial impact or refused nursing home care to avoid parting with the family home. Sensitivity and skill are required to negotiate these conversations and concerns while balancing the impact on the individual with the requirements of the organisation and systems within which one is operating.

Patients can often arrive at a hospice having had very difficult experiences in general hospitals where there was a lack of appropriate staff to manage their complex palliative care and symptom needs. There is therefore a very understandable reluctance to move on from somewhere providing a good level of palliative care. This can be compounded by concerns about the level of care and support available in the community.

Negative publicity about nursing homes and care agencies can combine with the financial constraints affecting the ability of nursing homes and care agencies to deliver the level of care they would wish to. This can be exacerbated by previous negative experiences of other family members and friends of the care system.

The increasing challenge of finding a nursing home that can provide a suitable level of palliative care nursing within travelling distance for family and friends and that has available places can be challenging. All this at the same time as continuing to visit the hospital or hospice, places additional strain on caregivers and families. Doing this alongside managing a job and/or childcare also creates additional stresses for the family. The strain on families can be significant and the role of the social worker is often focused on trying to enable patients' families to make difficult decisions within the resources available to meet the needs of the patient who may wish to die at home (Reith and Payne, 2009). There may be no appropriate places in nursing homes and the family are unable to manage someone dying at home. Promises may have been made to keep someone at home that prove impossible to keep and people need to be supported in managing this.

If a patient is insisting that a family member provides care for them it is important to consider the nature of the power balance in the relationship before the person became ill and the potential impact of this on the future wellbeing of both the individual and the caregiver. For example, there may be circumstances when there has been physical or emotional abuse within a relationship and the abuse can be exacerbated as the abuser struggles to adjust to a loss of control or the abused can suddenly find themselves in an unaccustomed position of power and control. While it can seem difficult to consider issues such as this in a palliative care context, often it is the social worker who is the team member with the experience and skills to make the most appropriate intervention, and safeguarding vulnerable adults is an important element of social work expertise.

When people experience times of crisis such as impending death, when they are likely to feel out of control and helpless, organisational pressures for efficiency can outweigh a holistic and person-centred approach, even for people receiving palliative care.

BEREAVEMENT CARE – THE ROLE OF THE SOCIAL WORKER

The provision of bereavement support can be a key role of the social worker in palliative care. Bereavement, can give rise to a wide range of needs – practical, financial, social, emotional and spiritual. There might be a need for information about loss and grief as well as family members wishing to pursue particular cultural practices who have a need for additional support to deal with the emotional and psychological impact of loss by death. In a small number of circumstances, there may be specific needs for mental health service intervention to cope with a mental health problem related to loss by death (Clukey, 2008).

Social workers can also be involved in providing support for parents in how to talk with children about what is happening, or they may work directly with children both pre- or post-bereavement.

Talking about and preparing for death when and if people feel able can be a significant part of the social work role (Reith and Payne, 2009). This can involve putting affairs in order and making plans, including, where appropriate, financial matters, making or revising a will, organising a power of attorney, considering management of their digital legacy (how any digital media accounts might be managed or the loss of photos, contacts or documents stored electronically that may be password protected (Digital Legacy Association, 2018). The author has also experienced situations where a person has been in great emotional distress about what will happen to a much loved pet when they are no longer able to care for them and have been greatly relieved when arrangements for a good future for the animal has been arranged via organisations such as the Cinnamon Trust.

BEREAVEMENT AFTERCARE

Many bereavement services in hospitals and hospices are partly staffed by volunteer counsellors and support workers who are involved in direct service provision (NICE, 2011). Social workers have much to offer from their professional perspective and make a significant contribution to the team effort in a spirit of collaboration and with confidence in their professional standpoint. A not uncommon problem after the death of a patient is the stress associated with paying for the funeral. The impact of funeral poverty can be financial, in the form of unmanageable debt, but it can also be emotional in the form of the distress, shame and the perceived stigma of not being able to provide a 'decent send-off' for someone we love (Fair Funerals, 2018).

The cost of funerals can be of huge concern to both patients and families and cause stress and concern at what would ideally be a time without this additional worry. People may also be unaware of what options are open to them with regard to funeral arrangements. This can both incur avoidable expense and mean that they may not have the type of funeral they would wish for. Social workers can play an important role in supporting discussion about individual needs and wishes and providing information and signposting. Sources of support and advice include the Natural Death Centre (www.naturaldeath.org.uk) and Quaker Social Action. People may also need support if they wish the deceased relative to be repatriated. If a person has no-one to organise their funeral the responsibility falls to the local authority. It is usually the role of the social worker to negotiate this alongside the designated worker from the local authority and try to ensure that the funeral is as personal as possible.

Different organisations like hospices provide a range of supportive services for families following death that include 'the day after death' meetings and memorial events where families of patients who have died are invited back to the hospice to share their feelings.

As previously discussed, social workers are experienced in facilitating difficult conversations about potentially painful subjects. Anticipatory grieving (grieving for a loss before it occurs) is thought to be a contributory protective factor in bereavement for some people (see Chapter 9).

Palliative care social workers are frequently involved in the provision of bereavement support services, often supervising a team of trained bereavement support volunteers (Graves, 2009). Social workers may also have additional qualifications in counselling and be able to provide support for people who need a greater level of support. An example is those whose experience of bereavement is much more intense than normal, lasts for much longer than usual or leads to the development of serious depression or other mental health problems (sometimes known as 'complicated grief' (see Chapter 9).

Hospitals have a limited number of bereavement aftercare services although these tend to be led by the spiritual care team and nurses (Costello, 1996). Complicated grief can develop in response to both the circumstances surrounding someone's death and the background against which it occurs. By providing appropriate pre-bereavement support the likelihood of complicated grief can be ameliorated (NICE, 2011). Specialist palliative care social workers can offer a wide variety of support to both the person and those who are important to them. For some bereaved family members, the experience of dying well can have a positive reaction on how bereaved people manage. Chapter 9 provides a comprehensive account of grief and bereavement and the role of practitioners in supporting the bereaved after death.

CONCLUSION

This chapter has considered the role of the social worker in palliative care and illustrated their often complex role using case studies of how social work intervention can and do make a difference to the palliative care journey. The chapter has described the nature of social work interventions in palliative care and above all highlighted the key skills of relationship-building and providing advice, support, empathy and compassion for people with life-limiting conditions, their families and carers. The chapter has discussed the social worker's role as a member of the multidisciplinary team and their unique role in supporting and contributing to the team. It has also considered the impact that death and dying can have on families and carers and, using authentic case studies, highlighted the role of the social worker. Social workers in palliative care provide support with emotional, legal, financial and practical issues. At the end of life they also help to organise and contribute to the support system that exists in hospices and hospitals for grieving patients and family members before and after death.

REFERENCES

Adams, R., Dominelli, L. and Payne, M. (eds) (2009) *Social Work: Themes, Issues and Critical Debates*. 3rd ed. Houndmills, Basingstoke: Palgrave Macmillan.

Agnew, A., Manktelow, R., Haynes, T. and Jones, L. (2011) 'Assessment practice in hospice settings: challenges for palliative care social workers.' *The British Journal of Social Work*, *41* (1): 111–30.

APCSW (2016) 'The Role Of A Palliative Care Social Worker.' Available at www.apcsw.org.uk/social-worker-role, accessed 13 July 2018.

Beresford, P., Adshead, L. and Croft, S. (2007) *Palliative Care, Social Work and Service Users: Making Life Possible*. London: Jessica Kingsley Publishers.

Beresford, P., Croft, S. and Adshead, L. (2008) '"We don't see her as a social worker": a service user case study of the importance of the social worker's relationship and humanity.' *British Journal of Social Work*, *38* (7): 1388–407.

Cagle, J.G. and Kovacs, P.J. (2009) 'Education: a complex and empowering social work intervention at the end of life.' *Health and Social Work*, *34* (1): 17–27.

Chaddock, R. (2016) 'Integrating early multi-disciplinary advance care planning into core social work practice: social workers' bread and butter.' *Journal of Social Work Practice*, *30* (2): 129–38.

Clukey, L. (2008) 'Anticipatory mourning: processes of expected loss in palliative care.' *International Journal of Palliative Nursing*, *14* (7): 316–25.

Costello, J. (1996) 'The emotional cost of palliative care.' *European Journal of Palliative Care*, *3* (4): 171–4.

Digital Legacy Association (2018) 'Sorting out your digital assets and digital legacy.' Available at: https://digitallegacyassociation.org, accessed July 2018.

Fair Funerals (2018) *What Is Funeral Poverty?* Available at http://fairfuneralscampaign.org.uk/content/what-funeral-poverty, accessed April 2018.

Graves, D. (2009) *Talking with Bereaved People: An Approach for Structured and Sensitive Communication*. London: Jessica Kingsley Publishers.

HM Government (2005) Mental Capacity Act, Chapter 9. HMSO.

Hughes, S., Firth, P. and Oliviere, D. (2014) 'Core competencies for palliative care social work in Europe: an EPAC white paper – part 1.' *European Journal of Palliative Care*, 21 (6): 300–5.

Munroe, B. (2005) 'Social work in palliative medicine', in G. Hanks, N.I. Cherny, N.A. Christakis, M. Fallon, S. Kaasa and R.K. Portenoy (eds) *Oxford Textbook of Palliative Medicine*. 3rd ed. Oxford: Oxford University Press.

National Institute for Clinical Excellence (NICE) (2004) *Improving Supportive and Palliative Care for Adults with Cancer*. CSG4. London: NICE.

National Institute for Clinical Excellence (NICE) (2011) *End of Life Care for Adults*. QS13. London: NICE.

National Institute for Clinical Excellence (NICE) (2017) *End of Life Care for People with Life- Limiting Conditions*. Available at https://pathways.nice.org.uk/pathways/end-of-life-care-for-people-with-life-limiting-conditions, accessed March 2017.

Reith, M. and Payne, M. (2009) *Social Work in End-of-Life and Palliative Care*. Bristol: Policy Press.

Scanlan, K. (2016) 'Psychosocial perspectives on end of life care.' *Journal of Social Work Practice*, 30 (2): 139–54.

Smith, S., Pugh, E. and McEvoy, M. (2012) 'Involving families in end of life care.' *Nursing Management*, 19 (4): 72–7.

FURTHER READING

APCSW (2016) Resources. Available at www.apcsw.org.uk/resources/, accessed 13 July 2018.

Cruse (2014) endorsed by the National Bereavement Alliance 'Bereavement Care Service Standards'.

Ellershaw, J.E., Dewar, S. and Murphy, D. (2010) 'Achieving a good death for all.' *British Medical Journal*, 341: c4861.

Gwyther, L.P., Altilio. T., Blacker S., Christ, G. et al. (2005) 'Social work competencies in palliative and end-of-life care.' *Journal of Social Work in End-of-Life & Palliative Care*, 1 (1): 87–120.

Hospice UK (2016) *A Low Priority? How Local Health and Care Plans Overlook the Needs of Dying People*. Available at www.hospiceuk.org/docs/default-source/ Policy-and-Campaigns/briefings-and-consultations-documents-and-files/hospiceuk_a_ low_priority_report.pdf, accessed 3 June 2018.

Kissanes, D.W. (2010) 'Bereavement', in G. Hanks, N.I. Cherny, N.A. Christakis, M. Fallon, S. Kaasa and R.K. Portenoy (eds) *Oxford Textbook of Palliative Medicine*. 4th ed. Oxford: Oxford Univesity Press.

Machin, L. (2014) *Working with Loss and Grief*. London: Sage.

Morrison, J. and Garland, E. (2004) 'Developing palliative care services in partnership.' *Cancer Nursing Practice*, 3 (3): 22–5.

Nielsen, M.K., Neergaard, M.A., Jensen, A.B., Bro, F. and Guldin, M.B. (2016) 'Do we need to change our understanding of anticipatory grief in caregivers? A systematic review of caregiver studies during end-of-life caregiving and bereavement.' *Clinical Psychology Review*, 44: 75–93.

Randall, F. and Downie, R.S. (2006) *The Philosophy of Palliative Care*. Oxford: Oxford University Press.

Relf, M., Machin, L. and Archer, N. (2010) *Guidance for Bereavement Needs Assessment in Palliative Care*. 2nd ed. Help the Hospices.

Scanlan, K. (2016) 'Psychological perspectives on palliative care', in G. Hanks, N.I. Cherny, N.A. Christakis, M. Fallon, S. Kaasa and R.K. Portenoy (eds) *Oxford Textbook of Palliative Medicine*. 4th ed. Oxford: Oxford University Press.

Sinclair, P. (2007) *Rethinking Palliative Care – A Social Role Valorisation Approach*. Bristol: Policy Press.

Spellman, A. (2014) *A Brief History of Death*. London: Reaktion Books.

9

GRIEF, BEREAVEMENT AND SPIRITUALITY

JOHN COSTELLO AND ANDREW BRADLEY

LEARNING OUTCOMES

- Develop a clear understanding of grief and bereavement related to palliative care
- Examine different understandings of spiritual care
- Evaluate the use of a model to enable spiritual care to be provided to patients at the end of life
- Consider the role of the practitioner in supporting patients and family members who are experiencing grief and conduct a bereavement risk assessment using a recognised tool

INTRODUCTION

This chapter focuses on the outcomes of palliative care at the end of life, the role of professionals in hospital and their role in helping patients and families manage grief and bereavement. Moreover, it looks at how practitioners can assess grief experiences and evaluate the risk of a person developing complicated or pathological grief using a risk assessment tool.

Once it becomes clear that the patient's condition is unlikely to respond to treatment a number of events can occur which can have a distressing impact on the patient and the family and give rise to uncertainty that may manifest itself in a spiritual way. The chapter looks at spirituality from the perspective of both the patient and members of the spiritual care team.

The take-home message of the chapter is that grief and bereavement are not illnesses, although in a small number of cases, grief, if not responded to properly, can become complicated and lead to mental health issues. As professional practitioners, it is important that, despite the uncomfortable and complex nature of grief, we become competent in our care for patients with a life-limiting illness. This involves providing them with high-quality palliative care and addressing their spiritual concerns. The challenge of providing effective psychosocial care is the ability of the practitioner to give high-quality care to the patient, but often at the same time offering emotional support to the family. To provide effective care requires practitioners to consider the outcomes of palliative care and to be prepared to support patients and families experiencing grief and bereavement (Costello, 2006). This chapter critically discusses grief and bereavement in the context of palliative care, considering differences between normal and abnormal grief. The chapter focuses on the role of the practitioner in supporting patients and family members experiencing grief and the interventions that can be made to alleviate distress.

BACKGROUND

In the UK over half a million people die each year, mostly in hospital (NeoLCP, 2011), with around 58 per cent of people dying in acute hospital settings (Gardner, 2012). Grief has been described as the experience of losing something or someone (Worden, 2009). In many cases the grief is due to human loss, the loss of a partner (conjugal grief), or the loss of a pet or in some cases intangible loss such as loss of freedom (when imprisoned), loss of an organ (after amputation or hysterectomy). Brown (2016) describes the loss of self that occurs when your normal pattern of self-identity or knowing who you are is changed, such as when a person is abused or when rape occurs. Many studies attest to the view that bereavement interventions, especially group-based interventions, have little impact on the experience of bereavement (Gauthier and Gagliese, 2012). Despite the lack of hard evidence, practitioners who effectively support those experiencing grief and bereavement are recognised as making a significant difference to individual suffering (De Souza and Pettifer, 2013). If asked, most people provide a basic explanation of the experience of grief, usually from personal experience, although few can describe its complexity. Patients and family members can experience loss at the end of life and this can take a number of different forms. Much depends on the person's previous experience of loss. This can be tangible, such as the death of a loved one, or intangible in the form of perhaps, amputation, house repossession or the loss of a relationship.

For practitioners, it is important to identify the links between what may be called the quality of the relationship and the experience of grief. There are a number of factors affecting the impact that loss will have including the loss history, the circumstances of the loss, the social network of the person and the kinds of strategies of coping that the individual adopts.

THE SOCIAL EXPERIENCE OF DYING

In the last two decades, the burgeoning literature on death and dying has revealed a number of papers, books and studies on what is referred to as 'good death'. Most focus on the social experience of death for the family with the occasional paper looking also at the impact of good and bad deaths on practitioners working in hospitals (Costello, 2006).

The concept of the good death is just that, it is an idea, an idealised way of considering how a person may wish to die and how these expectations can be met. Invariably good death scenarios are based on what is good for the patient. When teaching about types of death I often ask the audience how they would like to die. Suddenly, at home in bed; a heart attack that is sudden and quick with no pain; in your sleep; with dementia, etc. After having considered the different outcomes, many people settle on dying a quick, painless death without suffering. Sudden death causes tremendous grief and pain for those left behind. It makes sense therefore to consider for whom the death is good. For the patient, the family or even the staff that are providing end of life care.

Holdsworth (2015) points out that care providers play a much wider role in social aspects of care at the end of life than was previously considered and identified six themes associated with the good death, which included:

- one where care providers had a key role
- social engagement and connection to identity
- carer's confidence and ability to care
- preparation and awareness of death
- presentation of the patient at death
- support after death for protected grieving

GOOD AND BAD DEATHS

The concept of the good death is often associated with euthanasia or assisted dying. From an ethical perspective, nurses caring for people at the end of life describe good death as a powerful experience revealing rich insights into the way death is managed (Costello, 2004).

Good death scenarios according to De Souza and Pettifer (2013) are closely associated with the ability of the person to prepare for death. Moreover, they argue, good deaths may be characterised as ones where there is an effective level of communication between the nurse, the patient and the family. Baldwin and Woodhouse (2011) argue that a good death is a concept that each of us defines differently. Often, the patient may be aware that they are dying but in certain circumstances to protect the distress and the mobility of the patient, the patient is not aware of the diagnosis. Good deaths involve effective symptom control and nurses having an awareness of the person's spirituality and dignity. Moreover, it is important for nurses and patients to make joint decisions about the end of life, for example by the use of advanced care planning (ACP).

BAD DEATH SCENARIOS

Bad deaths, in contrast to good deaths, usually have a very negative effect on the family and the nurse. Bad deaths are often referred to as situations in which end of life and death was poorly managed, unexpected and caused stress to the patient, family and hospital staff (Brown, 2016). This contrasts with good death experiences as they may involve a lack of preparation, poor communication about the impending death, uncontrolled pain and other symptoms and a lack of understanding about the dying process. Bad deaths may exist as both individual experiences as well as organisational bad deaths whereby nurses and doctors collectively feel that the death was poorly managed (Costello, 2006).

Bad death scenarios can leave people (staff and family members) feeling guilty because of their perceived inability to influence the death. They can also contribute to the development of negative memories of the death. Bad death scenarios are remembered by nurses who recall patient experiences of distress, pain and suffering, and in many cases the family experienced anguish because they felt impotent to do anything about it. Here is a brief account of my mother's death from lung cancer when she was dying on a surgical ward. My sister was at my mother's bedside and became distressed because of the lack of pain control. Despite asking for pain relief several times, the nurses could not get the surgeon who was in theatre to return to the ward to prescribe pain relief. From sheer frustration my sister walked to the A&E department, found a junior doctor and persuaded him to come and see my mother who was dying. The doctor agreed, saw my mother and immediately prescribed morphine, which the nurses administered with good effect.

REFLECTIVE EXERCISE 9.1   GOOD AND BAD DEATHS

Good and bad deaths have an impact on us and influence the way we care. Take a moment to reflect on your own experiences of death and dying and the impact they had on you, both professionally and personally.

Make a list of what was good or bad about a death you have been involved in personally or professionally. Consider what made the death bad or good.

SPIRITUAL CARE

Often when we reflect on the impact of death it causes us to consider the spiritual aspects of life. Spirituality is often seen as a complex and sensitive issue which is hard to define but is a key issue when providing end of life care. Most hospitals and all hospices, in the UK and worldwide, have facilities for patients to receive spiritual care and support, especially around end of life. Hospitals throughout the world have people responsible for spiritual care provision, often in the form of members from the religious community. These chaplains form part of the spiritual care team providing religious support and spiritual/pastoral care.

The healthcare chaplain's religious support role is fairly straightforward; a patient has a religious need such as communion, confession or anointing, or access to sacred texts, or some kind of assistance with their prayers or rituals, and the chaplaincy team facilitates the meeting of that need, either through its own staff or volunteers, or through accessing appropriate religious support in the wider community. The value of a patient's religion in terms of coping with crisis includes regulation of health behaviours, provision of social resources, promotion of positive self-perceptions, provision of specific coping resources, generation of positive emotions, and additional hypothesised mechanisms such as the existence of a healing bioenergy (Cobb et al., 2012). However, it is recognised that religion does not always have a positive effect on patients' coping mechanisms (Cobb et al., 2012).

WHAT IS SPIRITUAL CARE?

Where people are struggling with life-limiting illness and challenging treatment, not to mention severe symptoms such as pain or nausea, spiritual care is often essential in terms of attending to such issues as meaning, purpose and hope. Concepts of spirituality and spiritual care have been the subject of endless debate and attempts at definition (Kellehear, 2000). Spirituality is perceived as a subjective experience that exists both within and outside traditional religious systems, which relates to the way in which people understand and live their lives in view of their sense of ultimate meaning and value (Cobb et al., 2012). Table 9.1 presents different perspectives from which spirituality can be understood, examples of what spiritual need may look like in the context of life-limiting illness according to these understandings, and then priorities in spiritual caregiving according to these needs.

In contemporary UK healthcare trusts, spiritual care teams often work closely with the palliative or supportive care teams in order to know when spiritual needs may arise with a patient and/or their carers. In the experience of both teams such needs tend to arise whenever there is a significant change in the patient's condition and/or prognosis – for example, when active treatment is withdrawn, or when the patient decides no longer to pursue such treatment. Spiritual assessment is also a matter of course when the patient is identified as being in the last days of life, according to NICE guidance (2017). It is at these times of significant change that the team needs to ensure that a spiritual assessment has taken place. A useful guide here is the Macmillan Holistic Needs Assessment model, a diagnostic tool that takes account of physical, practical, family/relationship, emotional, spiritual and lifestyle concerns (Macmillan Cancer Support, 2012).

Table 9.1 illustrates how spiritual need/care go far beyond religious support, though the two may sometimes intersect. But for non-religious patients and their families there may well be an issue around such spiritual care being

Table 9.1 Different perspectives on spirituality

Spirituality	Spiritual need	Spiritual care
Knowledge (especially ideographic)	Recognition of the uniqueness of the patient's experience of their illness 'This is *my* cancer'	Empathy Active, patient-centred listening
Personhood	The need for identity 'Who am I?'	Life review Encouraging connection with significant others
Belief	Investment of trust in human or divine agent	Reassurance
Hope	'To sing sweetly in the face of a storm'	Enabling patient to set realistic goals Mindfulness
Meaning making	Making sense in times of crisis	Normalising and attending to existential distress
Compassion	Knowing somebody cares	'The art of compassionate presence' (Taylor C. and Walker S., Cobb et al., 2012: Ch. 20) focus on manner of caring as well as outcomes
Dignity	A sense of spiritual peace (Sinclair S. and Chochinov H.M., Cobb et al., 2012: Ch. 21)	Accurate spiritual assessment for both patient and carers
Cure and healing	Wholeness – the acceptance of one's sacredness in all circumstances (Balducci L. and Modditt H.L., Cobb et al., 2012: Ch. 22)	Value history, including personal goals and preferences (Balducci L. and Modditt H.L., Cobb et al., 2012: Ch. 22)
Suffering	Spiritual pain – meaninglessness, worthlessness, loneliness or emptiness (Ferrell B. and Del Ferraro C., Cobb et al., 2012: Ch. 23)	Creating meaning, facilitating the grieving of losses, emphasising continuity between past and future (Ferrell B. and Del Ferraro C., Cobb et al., 2012: Ch. 23)
Ritual	Giving significance to life changes	Words or actions that facilitate the crossing of thresholds (Davies D.J., Cobb et al., 2012: Ch. 24)

delivered by spiritual caregivers from religious traditions, however flexible they may be. At the time of writing, there is a vigorous debate going on in NHS chaplaincy circles: how might such people have equal access to a spiritual care service essentially provided by religious people (i.e. chaplains from religious traditions)? One strategy could be to deploy chaplains and volunteers from a variety of faith and belief backgrounds, including humanist. This raises the question of what might non-religious spiritual care look like, not just for the spiritual care team, but for other health professionals seeking to engage authentically with spiritual need in a non-religious framework?

UNDERSTANDING SPIRITUAL CARE

Understanding and responding to the spiritual needs of others can be a difficult and daunting task for many practitioners working in palliative care.

Kellehear's work (2000) is instructive here, as he posits a threefold model of spiritual need which brings some clarity to the plethora of spiritual care/need definitions. It is based largely on the 'meaning making' understanding of spirituality (Cobb et al., 2012) through which human beings transcend hardship and suffering. According to Kellehear, human beings in crisis situations will seek meaning and transcendence on three different levels: situational, moral/biographical and religious. The need for situational transcendence in the supportive care setting springs from the immediacy of a situation such as developing symptoms, the impact of being admitted into a clinical environment, and facing one's mortality, and the response to such needs is something every non-religious spiritual caregiver can deliver. This response may include companionship, listening, affirmation, advocacy and presence.

At the second moral/biographical level of seeking transcendence, issues may emerge such as the need for forgiveness, reconciliation or closure, especially as one's life draws to an end. Except in the area of prayer, which is sometimes a need expressed at this level (Kellehear, 2000) such issues need not and should not be addressed by 'religious dogma' or 'theological opinion', unless expressly requested by the patient, and non-religious spiritual caregiving is still pertinent here – for example, in the form of helping with life review or connecting with significant relationships.

At the third religious level, a patient's past or current religious practice may come to the fore, with attendant needs such as forgiveness, healing, grace or strength from a divine or supernatural dimension. Kellehear argues strongly that responses to needs at this level should not be watered down by caregivers – for example, for fear of being seen to proselytise – but opportunities must be sought out for sacred rites, and religious visitation and discussion, presumably from appropriate religious caregivers (Kellehear, 2000).

An example from recent experience illustrates the pertinence of this threefold model of levels of spiritual need (see Case study 9.1).

CASE STUDY 9.1   PAULA

Paula was referred to the spiritual care team by the supportive care multidisciplinary team (MDT) as supportive care nurses had noticed that a religious medallion from Lourdes (a Roman Catholic site of pilgrimage) seemed especially important to her. She had also used spiritual language when expressing pain and distress. Over the space of about a month, the team was involved with this patient on seven occasions. It transpired that she was Roman Catholic but had not attended church for some years. However, she told us that she prayed, especially with reference to her medallion, and that recently she found herself praying often for people she had met in a local day hospice which she attended.

Initially Paula was resistant to any advance care planning, mainly because she did not want to upset her son, but as her prognosis worsened, and she was referred to a hospice for ongoing care, this changed dramatically. She began planning in earnest for a non-religious ceremony followed by a burial.

The input of the spiritual care team happened in four ways. First, through listening to the patient's story, the team was able to help her express her sense of grief and loss in terms of independence, routine and lifestyle. Second, we gave her a printed in-house resource which is a tool for self-reflection in non-religious language as an aid to reducing her anxiety. Third, there was one conversation with the patient's parents, in which they were able to be reassured that their daughter's spiritual needs were being met – this was important to them. According to Kellehear's model, all of this was meeting situational spiritual need.

Fourth, on one occasion there was a significant conversation about death and the afterlife. This conversation was initiated in the context of talking about funeral plans, when Paula asked me, 'You must have seen a lot of people dying – what's it like?' I spoke about my experience of being around death and dying, and Paula told me she felt reassured. I encouraged her to ask her supportive care nurses if she felt she wanted to get more information about the process of dying.

Then came a second question, and this was more of a surprise. 'I'd like to think I'm going to be with my loved ones – does that actually happen, or is it something you just carry with you, like in your head?'

I asked for clarification, and understood that Paula was wondering whether meeting with departed loved ones was in any way 'real', or was it something going on in one's consciousness in the last moments of life.

Again, referring to Kellehear's model, Paula at this point shifted from a situational to a moral/biographical level of spiritual need, and again I shared my own experience of end of life situations, and how anecdotally at least some patients and their carers had spoken of a sense of loved ones departed coming close. I also spoke about the conversations I had been privileged to hold with people who had had NDEs (near death experiences), and the common themes of light, and a sense of peace and unconditional love they had expressed; one patient spoke about being in a place where she felt she utterly 'belonged'. On a philosophical level, we agreed that even though experience and indeed many faiths and beliefs talk about some sort of afterlife, no-one really knows what happens at and after death, and that even if the afterlife only takes place in our consciousness, this does not necessarily make it any less 'real'.

Although Paula had a Roman Catholic upbringing, I decided not to refer overly to the doctrine of her childhood faith, as she had not mentioned it. With reference to Kellehear's model, her need remained on a moral/biographical level, and not a religious one. I question whether any non-religious spiritual caregiver would have been able to engage on this level without some formal training in theology and philosophy; however, even someone without such training should have been able to bring to bear those situational level skills such as good listening and reassurance, as long as there was practical capacity in terms of patient contact time.

The patient concluded by saying, 'I don't feel I can really discuss these things with my family, because I don't want to upset them, so I'm really glad I've been able to ask you.' Whatever the capacity of the professional spiritual caregiver, the importance of a less involved, more objective listener than family carers, especially in terms of spiritual questioning, should never be underestimated or taken away from people facing their last days of life.

GRIEF, BEREAVEMENT AND PALLIATIVE CARE

GRIEF MODELS AND THEORIES

There are a number of grief theories, which emanate from the seminal work of Freud (1957 [1917]), through to the work of John Bowlby (1980) in the UK, William Worden (2009) in the USA, Colin Murray Parkes (1972) in the UK, Stroebe and Schut (1999) in Germany and Klass et al. (1996) in the USA. There are of course many other contributors such as Wortman and Silver (1989), who have looked at loss and coping strategies, and with others who have made a substantive contribution to the debate and research on grief and bereavement. However, in this chapter I have attempted to focus on most well-known models and theories. At the end of the chapter Table 9.2 summarises and illustrates the key theorists and their contribution. Interestingly, the work of Elizabeth Kubler Ross (1969) was not in the list because she said her work was not a grief theory despite it being taught in British nurse education as a theory of grief. Her famous five stages – anger, denial, bargaining, depression and acceptance – are familiar to many nurses (even the sixth stage of hope). Explanations of grief need to take note of its cultural significance and how different cultures respond to death, especially as the world is rapidly developing into a cultural melting pot (Firth, 2001). Grief theories may be categorised according to their focus. Those from the more psychotherapeutic end of the spectrum (e.g. Freud, 1957 [1917]; Parkes, 1972; and Worden, 2009) see grief as an expression of feelings and behaviours that occur in stages or phases. Individuals develop through grief by encountering emotional tasks referred to as grief work. These stage- and phase-based models enable us to identify the stage experienced by the mourner. In this way, it may be argued that the grief model rather than describing grief instead prescribes grief (i.e. you hear people say they are in denial or going through anger).

NORMAL GRIEF

Grief may be seen as the emotional dimension of loss, and bereavement the social fact of loss. Theories and models of grief that include stages and phases tend to portray a linear pattern which in the end have a positive outcome. Kubler-Ross's (1969) five-stage model is a good example where after anger, denial, bargaining and depression comes acceptance. Adopting this way of thinking about grief models, it is possible to see a sense of hope in the stage-based approaches to understanding grief. The stages or phases as they have been described represent the grief work which is primarily understood to be the emotional component of grief where the mourner works through their grief. This emotional transition is influenced by the circumstances of the death, the relationship of attachment to the deceased and the mourners' supporting networks. However, should the mourner, for whatever reason, fail or become (emotionally) stuck in their grief work, then, according to the grief work approach, complications can arise, such as depression.

STAGE- AND PHASE-BASED MODELS

These theories referred to by Payne et al. (2011) as developmental theories have their origins in the work of Freud (1957 [1917]) who identified differences between depression and grief. Freud's thesis was that people developed an emotional attachment to others and this emotional energy was a form of love. Parkes (1972) later pointed out in relation to grief intensity that the greater the love the greater the grief when loss occurred. However, the mourner wishes to relinquish the emotional bond with the deceased and at the same time stay attached because of the strength of the bond. Mourners therefore experience 'grief work', as they strive to detach from the bond with the deceased. The bereaved need to accept the reality of the loss and emotionally move on or, as Worden points out, emotionally relocate. For those models that subscribe to what Stroebe and Schut (1999) call the 'grief work hypothesis', it is necessary for the mourner to break the emotional bond with the deceased in order to achieve a successful bereavement outcome. They do this by experiencing a number of stages or phases.

DIFFERENT APPROACHES TO UNDERSTANDING GRIEF

Parkes's (1972) seminal work on phases of grief utilised Freud's earlier work as well as contributions from John Bowlby's research on attachment (1980). Parkes's phase theory focused on the resolution of grief via a process of four major overlapping phases of realisation, whereby the mourner comes to terms with the fact of loss by first experiencing *shock and numbness*; in phase 2, *yearning and searching*, they may refuse or deny the reality of the loss. They may try searching for the deceased, but once it becomes clear that the deceased will not return, the mourner experiences feelings of anger and frustration. In phase 3, *disorganisation and despair*, the mourner becomes easily distracted, lacks concentration and may experience depression. At this phase, the mourner may come to the realisation that the deceased is not coming back, leading to confusion and uncertainty about their future. Finally, in the fourth phase, *reorganisation and recovery*, the mourner may come to terms with their loss and take steps to carry on with life.

TASKS MODEL (WORDEN, 2009)

In a similar process to Parkes, Worden, an American psychoanalyst, takes a more active approach arguing that the bereaved must emotionally work through four major tasks (with help from a counsellor if required):

- Task 1: Accept the reality of the loss
- Task 2: Manage/process the pain of loss/grief
- Task 3: Adjust to life without the deceased
- Task 4: Emotional relocation (moving on)

Lindemann (1944), an American psychiatrist, developed an approach similar to others that included acceptance of the loss, adjustment to a life without the deceased and the formation of new relationships. Kubler Ross's stages of grief have a lot of similarities with the psychiatric/psychoanalytical approaches, although there is no directive to work through grief and all stages may be seen as reactions to the news of a cancer diagnosis as the original text made clear. All of the key theorists have modified and adapted their original work as a result of new research and ideas and the descriptions given may be seen as a core baseline representation of the complexity of their theories.

DUAL PROCESS MODEL (STROEBE AND SCHUT, 1999)

The dual process model is an explanation of how the bereaved cope with many and often conflicting issues that arise when someone dies. Essentially it is an abstract way of illustrating how bereaved people come to terms with significant loss. However, it can be used in relation to spousal and other losses. The model attempts to make sense of the competing stressors associated with bereavement, cognitive strategies related to adapting to loss (grief work), by illustrating this as a *dynamic process of oscillation*. The two main forces are the loss-oriented (grief work focused) and the restorative-oriented issues associated with dealing with necessary life changes, with everyday life experiences being part of both processes as illustrated in Figure 9.1. This makes the dual process model unique from other grief theories.

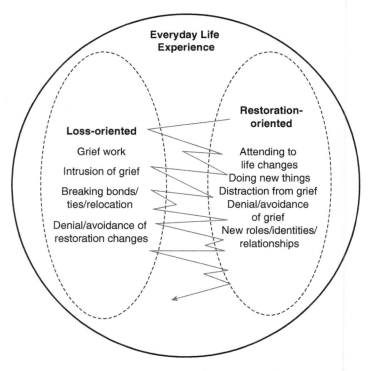

Figure 9.1   Dual process model Stroebe and Schut (1999)

CONTINUING BONDS MODEL (KLASS ET AL., 1996)

The continuing bond concept focuses almost in the opposite way of the grief work hypothesis. Instead of breaking the emotional bond with the deceased, the bereaved person and the deceased continue to have an enduring spiritual relationship (Klass et al., 1996). This theory, which interestingly is supported by writers such as Parkes, identifies that in some cases not breaking the emotional bond can have beneficial effects. In the case of older people, Stephen (2012) points out that continuing bond relationships tend to be experienced by older bereaved people, who she argues should be given time to develop explanations and understanding of the death. Moreover, Field et al. (2003) suggest that in relation to conjugal bereavement, participants who reported high levels of relationship satisfaction prior to death demonstrated a corresponding propensity to develop continuing bond relationships, which endured for many years after death. Table 9.2 lists the key authors and titles of their seminal work on grief and bereavement.

SUPPORTIVE INTERVENTIONS

One useful way of assessing the impact of loss and helping the person is by doing a simple exercise called a loss line (see Figure 9.2). Loss lines involve asking what previous losses the griever has experienced, be they tangible or intangible, and illustrating them on a piece of paper in the form of horizontal lines against a vertical line. The horizontal lines denote the emotional intensity of loss.

In Figure 9.2 you can see that the death of my mother when I was aged 26 was a huge loss. Loss lines can help provide a basis for interaction about the loss experience and what grief means. In the example, age is used to identify when the loss occurred. At the age of 11, I lost my dog (Beauty), I had her from being a puppy at the age of six and she was put to sleep. My mother died when I was 26, it was a

Table 9.2   Summary of Grief Theories

Name of author	Year	Title of book/paper
Lindemann	1944	Symptomatology and management of acute grief
Freud	1957 [1917]	Mourning and melancholia
Kübler-Ross	1969	On death and dying
Parkes	1972	Studies of grief in adult life
Wortman and Silver	1989	Coping with irrevocable loss
Worden	1991	Grief counselling and grief therapy
Klass et al.	1996	Continuing bonds: New understandings of grief
Stroebe and Schut	1999	Dual process model of coping with bereavement

huge loss for me as I was a practising nurse at the time, and it was a bad death in many ways. At the age of 31, my father died, at home with the family and despite it being a sad time, it was also a good death, hence the shorter horizontal line.

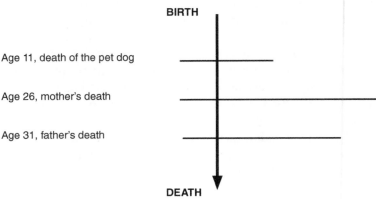

Figure 9.2   Loss lines

EXERCISE 9.2   LOSS LINES

Try the loss lines exercise yourself and reflect on your personal loss experiences. Don't forget to include any loss that had an impact on you, not just death. Try to consider what support you were given (or not) and how well you coped. Was or is there any residual emotion still lingering about the loss?

Most people experience loss as a natural healthy process without developing any specific problems, although assessing those key factors that can lead to complicated grief is important (Hawton, 2007). Assessing the impact of loss can be very challenging and nurses are sometimes well placed to assess likely grief reactions because of their close contact with family and friends of the deceased. It is important to identify if a recently bereaved person is adapting to their new role adequately. The risk, as Alexander and Klein (2012) point out, is that some people can develop complicated grief reactions also referred to as pathological grief, chronic grief or abnormal grief. Alexander and Klein (2012) regard the following criteria as constituting concern about grief becoming pathological.

COMPLICATED GRIEF REACTIONS

One way of assessing the impact of the loss on family members and others is to use a bereavement risk assessment tool. These are more often used by nurses and social workers in hospices, although they can be used effectively in other settings such as hospital wards. The tool commonly used was developed from the seminal work of Parkes in 1990. The aim of the tool is to assist professionals with the assessment of those behavioural predictors that can be picked up around the time of death which may adversely influence the feelings of the bereaved family and could lead to complicated grief. The risk assessment includes collating an initial set of biographical data followed by seven short sections, each with five or six items. The scoring is based on a scale of 1 to 5, with 1 being the lowest score. All scoring 4 or 5 in any category with an asterisk requires follow-up. The tool allows you to assess the severity of grief and pick up on specific reactions as being abnormal.

BEREAVEMENT RISK ASSESSMENT

The bereavement risk assessment tool may be used to identify factors which may complicate the grief of the key person(s) experiencing bereavement. These commonly include:

- Severity of symptoms/reactions
- Duration of symptoms/reactions
- Delayed onset of symptoms/reactions
- Level of dysfunction related to home and work life

When conducting an assessment in relation to the severity of the responses, it is necessary to consider the relationship of attachment, the circumstances of the death and the social network that the bereaved can utilise. The assessment of specific reactions as normal or abnormal needs to be considered in the context of what Alexander and Klein (2012) identify as criteria for establishing differences between normal and abnormal grief reaction. The amount and type of support given to the bereaved can be as simple as inviting the families back to the ward for an annual get together of families who have experienced loss (see Costello, 1996). These ward-based memorial-type events work well in hospices and certain long stay settings where families have a chance to memorialise the dead, share experiences and gain comfort from being amongst others.

In summary, bereavement support takes a variety of forms. In some cases, the bereaved will be thankful for practical help to alleviate the burden of doing day-to-day tasks they cannot face. In other cases, a listening ear is required to enable them to offload their emotional turmoil in order to make sense of the confusion often created by loss.

CONCLUSION

This chapter focused attention on the need to develop a clear understanding of loss, grief and bereavement in their different forms both theoretically and practically related to palliative care at the end of life. It also considers the complex issue of spirituality and how nurses and others can provide spiritual support for the patient and family members at the end of life. The chapter looked at dying experiences and how good and bad death concepts can impact on patients, families and health practitioners. Moreover, the chapter has considered the role of the practitioner in supporting patients and family members who experience spiritual pain and loss and how a risk assessment can be made of their bereavement in order to avoid grief becoming complicated.

REFERENCES

Alexander, D. and Klein, S. (2012) 'Mental health trauma and bereavement', in P. Wimpenny and J. Costello (eds), *Grief, Loss and Bereavement*. London: Routledge.

Baldwin, M.A. and Woodhouse, J. (2011) 'Good death', in M.A. Baldwin and J. Woodhouse (eds), *Key Concepts in Palliative Care*. London: Sage.

Bowlby, J. (1980) *Attachment and Loss: Loss, Sadness, and Depression*. New York: Basic Books.

Brown, M. (2016) *Palliative Care in Nursing and Health Care*. London: Sage.

Cobb, M.R., Puchalski, C.M. and Rumbold, B. (2012) *Oxford Textbook of Spirituality in Healthcare*. Oxford: Oxford University Press.

Costello, J. (1996) 'Acknowledging loss: reflections on bereavement.' *Elderly Care*, 8, (4): 35–6.

Costello, J. (2004) *Nursing the Dying Patient: Caring in Different Contexts*. London: Palgrave.

Costello, J. (2006) '"Dying well": Nurses' experiences of good and bad deaths in hospital.' *Journal of Advanced Nursing*, 54, (5): 1–8.

De Souza, J. and Pettifer, A. (2013) *End-of-Life Nursing Care*. London: Sage.

Field, N.P., Gal-Oz, E. and Bonanno, G.A. (2003) 'Continuing bonds and adjustment at five years after the death of a spouse.' *Journal of Consulting and Clinical Psychology*, 71, (1): 110–17.

Firth, S. (2001) 'Hindu death and mourning rituals: the impact of geographic mobility', in J. Hockey, J. Katz and N. Small (eds) *Grief, Mourning and Death Ritual*. Buckingham: Open University Press.

Freud, S. (1957 [1917]) 'Mourning and melancholia', in J. Strachey (ed., nd translation), *The Standard Edition of the Complete Psychological Works of Sigmund Freud*. Vol. 14. New York: Basic Books.

Gardner, D.B. (2012) 'Quality in life and death: can we have the conversations?' *Nursing Economics*, 30 (4): 224–6, 232.

Gauthier, L.R. and Gagliese, L. (2012) 'Bereavement interventions, end-of-life cancer care, and spousal well-being: a systematic review.' *Clinical Psychology, Science and Practice*, 19, (1): 72–92.

Hawton, J. (2007) 'Complicated grief after bereavement: psychological interventions may be effective.' *British Medical Journal*, 334 (7601): 962–3.

Holdsworth, L.M. (2015) 'Bereaved carers' accounts of the end of life and the role of care providers in a "good death": a qualitative study.' *Palliative Medicine*, 29 (9): 834–41.

Kellehear, A. (2000) 'Spirituality and palliative care: a model of needs.' *Palliative Medicine*, 14: 149–55.

Klass, D., Silverman, P. and Nickman, S. (eds) (1996) *Continuing Bonds: New Understandings of Grief*. Washington DC: Taylor & Francis.

Kubler-Ross, E. (1969) *On Death and Dying*. London: Macmillan.

Lindemann, E. (1944) 'Symptomatology and management of grief.' *American Journal of Psychiatry*, *151* (6 Suppl.): 155–60.

Macmillan Cancer Support (2012) *National Cancer Survivorship Initiative: Concerns Checklist*. https://be.macmillan.org.uk/Downloads/ResourcesForHSCPs/AboutMacmillansServices/MAC13689IdentifyingconcernsPadHR.pdf, accessed October 2018

National End of Life Care Programme (NeoLCP) (2011) *When a Person Dies: Guidance for Professionals on Developing Bereavement Services*. London: NHS.

National Institute for Health and Care Excellence (NICE) (2017) *End of Life Care for People with Life-Limiting Conditions*. Available at https://pathways.nice.org.uk/pathways/end-of-life-care-for-people-with-life-limiting-conditions, accessed March 2017.

Parkes, C. (1972) *Bereavement: Studies of grief in adult life*. London: Tavistock.

Payne, S., Lloyd–Williams, M. and Kennedy, V. (2011) 'Bereavement care and hope', in M. Lloyd-Williams (ed.) *Psychosocial Issues in Palliative Care*. 2nd ed. Oxford: Oxford University Press.

Stephen, A. (2012) 'Bereavement and older people', in P. Wimpenny and J. Costello (eds), *Grief, Loss and Bereavement*. London: Routledge.

Stroebe, M. and Schut, H. (1999) 'The dual process model of coping with bereavement: rationale and description.' *Death Studies*, *23* (3): 197–224.

Worden, W. (2009) *Grief Counselling and Grief Therapy: A Handbook for the Mental Health Practitioner*. 4th ed. New York: Springer.

Wortman, C.B. and Silver, R.C. (1989) 'The myth of coping with loss.' *Journal of Consulting and Clinical Psychology*, *57* (3): 349–57.

FURTHER READING

Akner, L.F. (1994) *How to Survive the Loss of a Parent: A Guide for Adults*. New York: William Morrow.

Brown, M. (2016) *Palliative Care in Nursing and Health Care*. London: Sage.

General Medical Council (2010) *Treatment and Care towards the End of Life: Good Practice in Decision-Making*. Available at www.gmc-uk.org/static/documents/content/Treatment_and_care_towards_the_end_of_life_-_English_1015.pdf, accessed 11 April 2017.

Lewis, C.S. (1961) *A Grief Observed*. London: Faber and Faber.

Payne, S., Horn, S. and Relf, M. (1999) *Loss and Bereavement*. Buckingham: Open University Press.

Payne, S., Seymour, J. and Ingleton C. (eds) (2008) *Palliative Care Nursing: Principles and Evidence for Practice*. 2nd ed. Buckingham: Open University Press.

Wimpenny, P. and Costello, J. (eds) *Grief, Loss and Bereavement*. London: Routledge.

10

ETHICAL DILEMMAS IN PALLIATIVE CARE

ANNE-MARIE RAFTERY AND CAROLE FARRELL

LEARNING OUTCOMES

- Engage in debate about the types of ethical dilemmas commonly occurring in palliative care contexts
- Consider ways of explaining challenges caused by a patient's lack of competence to make decisions about their healthcare
- Identify appropriate ways of disclosing sensitive information to patients and families
- Discuss ways of dealing with difficulties associated with collusion

Palliative care, especially at the end of life, raises numerous ethical issues. This chapter highlights several key ethical issues that often present when a patient has a life-limiting condition, including Do not attempt resuscitation orders (DNAR), advance care planning (ACP), disclosing sensitive information about diagnosis (breaking bad news), collusion and patient competence. The chapter highlights the experiences of patients and family who respond in different ways to ethical issues.

INTRODUCTION

Ethics in palliative and end of life care has arguably increased in complexity in recent years, largely due to an increase in technology and biological treatments. This creates challenges for healthcare professionals when balancing patient/family expectations and concerns, such as uncertainty about diagnosis and prognosis, information needs and treatment/supportive care options (Hagerty et al., 2005).

The role of healthcare professionals, guided by the Hippocratic oath 'to cure sometimes, to relieve often and to comfort always', given there are often few absolutes or certainties, alongside the use of good communication and compassion, is perhaps even more pressing. Faull and Blankley (2015) suggest this requires the healthcare team to weigh up carefully the appropriateness of three considerations:

- Will investigations or treatments be appropriate and enhance quality of life?
- Do the benefits outweigh the burdens?
- Are they certain not to bring suffering?

Yet if we apply these considerations – to the appropriateness of investigations, for example – the benefits and burdens are not always clear, and may be compounded by uncertainty and different perspectives, such as what is considered 'acceptable', 'quality of life' or 'suffering'.

Ethics is the moral principle that governs a person's behaviour or the conducting of an activity (Oxford English Dictionary, 2017). We can therefore see that ethics in healthcare can pose real dilemmas and difficulties, not only for the patient, but for the family and clinician alike.

There are broadly two main theories of ethical theory relevant to healthcare, that of consequentialism (utilitarianism) and deontology.

CONSEQUENTIALISM

Consequentialism is where the consequences of each action and possible course promoting best consequences are considered. The most influential consequentialist approach was utilitarianism in the 19th century, made famous by John Stuart Mill and Jeremy Bentham with Bentham's well-known phrase 'the greatest good for the greatest number' (Beauchamp and Childress, 2001).

DEONTOLOGY

Deontology is the duties that we have to one another. This can resonate strongly with healthcare professionals who endeavour to promote wellbeing and avoid harm, often termed 'duty based ethics'. The most influential deontologist in the 18th century was Immanuel Kant (Beauchamp and Childress, 2001).

ETHICAL FRAMEWORK

The four 'pillars of medical ethics' – autonomy, non-maleficence, beneficence and justice (see Table 10.1) – often present when patients have life-limiting conditions. Using a practical framework (Beauchamp and Childress, 2001) can provide a useful application to working ethics, given the complexities and dilemmas for patient care within medicine and nursing.

Table 10.1   The four 'pillars of medical ethics'

AUTONOMY	Patients' right to make their own decisions
BENEFICENCE	One ought to act and do good
NON-MALEFICENCE	Do no harm (enshrined by the Hippocratic oath)
JUSTICE	To treat patients in a similar manner (equity)

Using a case study and clinical examples, this chapter will highlight the experiences of patients and families who respond in different ways to ethical issues, emphasising complex issues of communication and collusion. The main premise of the four core ethical principles will be assumed, given their widespread use in clinical practice. This will facilitate discussions around ethical issues, while acknowledging the limitations of pure ethical principles.

These four principles are considered prima facie in that they stand alone in a non-hierarchical fashion and are considered independently of one another (Beauchamp and Childress, 2001). Whether this in fact plays out in clinical practice is open to debate and will be considered throughout this chapter.

CASE STUDY 10.1   SARAH

(The case study is based on several patients' experiences)

Sarah, a 39 year old woman with a stage IIIC primary peritoneal cancer, was admitted with symptoms of bowel obstruction (faecal vomiting and abdominal colic) while undergoing her fifth cycle of palliative chemotherapy (carboplatin/taxol). She was diagnosed several months prior following emergency surgery for bowel perforation, which resulted in an ileo-cutaneous fistula and stoma formation. Since then she had required parenteral nutrition.

A restaging CT scan during this admission unfortunately revealed disease progression, with extensive serosal disease, lung and liver metastases with multiple sites of bowel obstruction.

Sarah stated clearly that she did not wish to know the CT scan results unless they revealed 'good news'. Her husband agreed with her request and Sarah agreed that he could be involved in any clinical discussions. She continually repeated the same statement when efforts were made to discuss the CT scan: 'I have to live for my children' and was insistent that further chemotherapy be continued. Sarah also refused to discuss her future care needs, including a venting gastrostomy for symptom control.

The community-based teams expressed concerns regarding her discharge home since she declined all community support and hospice admission for symptom control/end of life care prior to this admission.

This situation raised ethical concerns and dilemmas for clinicians, including whether to continue chemotherapy and parenteral nutrition since she was approaching the last few months of life and did not want to fully engage in any honest discussions around risks/benefits of treatment and quality of life.

When oral nutritional intake deteriorates, this can raise ethical tensions around when (and if) to consider alternative methods of artificial feeding. This requires ethical principles of beneficence and non-maleficence alongside futility and resource allocation, to guide this decision-making process (Beauchamp and Childress, 2001; National Cancer Institute, 2013).

The potential benefits must be carefully considered (Baracos, 2013). A Cochrane review concludes that there is 'a lack of evidence to make recommendations for practice in palliative patients' (Good et al., 2014). Evidence on the role of parenteral feeding in advanced cancer is also poor given the lack of randomised controlled trials and possible ethical issues around randomising patients with advanced cancer to parenteral versus non-parenteral feeding.

Conversely, The European Society for Clinical Nutrition and Metabolism (ESPEN) guidance stipulates that parenteral feeding should only be used for those with a non-functioning gut or where access to the gastrointestinal tract for enteral feeding is not possible; for example, bowel obstruction or intestinal failure (Bozzetti et al., 2009). Furthermore, it is also important to consider the appropriateness of continuing any artificial nutrition intervention if it has already been started. The Royal College of Physicians (2010) state that clear reasons must be identified for such withdrawal, alongside discussions with the patient, family and healthcare professional. Cultural differences should be addressed, particularly if they differ from medical opinion (General Medical Council, 2010).

NON-MALEFICENCE

The aim of non-maleficence is to avoid or do no harm, yet decisions around non-maleficence and medical futility appear to have a high media profile. One example is the emotive case of baby Charlie Guard who had irreparable brain damage from a mitochondrial genetic disorder. This case highlighted complex discussions around medical futility and quality of life, and the dignity, compassion and care by Charlie's parents and healthcare professionals, including a need to prevent further suffering.

JUSTICE

Justice is to treat patients fairly and includes the fair distribution of resources, limitations and competing demands.

Yet in the current financial climate, the NHS cannot meet all these ethical values due to finite budgets and restricted resources. This brings into sharp focus the notion that treatment at all costs is not necessarily the right course of action, which was identified in the National Confidential Enquiry for Patient Outcomes and Deaths (NCEPOD) report (2008). NCEPOD urged oncologists to ask patients about advance decisions they may wish to make to promote early decision making by senior clinicians, suggesting that patients facing incurable cancer are 'extremely vulnerable'. The report also states that lines between informing, persuading and manipulating can become blurred. Therefore, obtaining informed consent can be difficult when well-meaning family members and clinicians may cloud decision-making processes and supersede the patient's wishes. The report also emphasised difficulties about achieving a balance between honesty and maintaining hope and optimism when faced with an incurable, progressive illness. However, it is important to avoid futile treatments and patient harm.

Within this context, a treatment is considered futile if a response is physiologically impossible, if it is non-beneficial or unlikely to produce the desired benefit. The 'elephant in the room' is often economics – for example, the cost of intensive care facilities for people with advancing cancer.

AUTONOMY

Autonomy is a person's right to make their own decisions, which is a fundamental part of humanity, setting us apart from animals. There are many different accounts of what constitutes autonomy (Dworkin, 1988; O'Neill, 2002), although Immanuel Kant and John Stuart Mill have shaped the interpretation of autonomy throughout the centuries (Beauchamp and Childress, 2001).

For Kant, autonomy is an expression of rationality that makes us worthy of respect, because we are autonomous and capable of rationally determining our own 'ends'. Thus, autonomy has intrinsic value and forms part of personal development, even during the last months of life (Beauchamp and Childress, 2001).

Gillon (1985) suggests that autonomy is 'self-rule', thus having autonomy enables us to deliberate and make our own decisions and respect for other people's autonomy becomes a moral obligation. However, there must be equal respect for everyone's autonomy at the same time, which is difficult to achieve in complex situations.

KANT'S INTERPRETATION OF AUTONOMY

In this section, Kant's interpretation of autonomy and the implications for palliative and end of life care will be outlined with reference to Sarah's case. Kant described respect for autonomy as 'treating others as ends in themselves and never merely as means'; which is considered a 'categorical imperative' (Gillon, 1985), which means that to violate someone's autonomy would be treating that person as a 'means to an end' (Beauchamp and Childress, 2001).

Therefore, for Kant, a decision is autonomous if it is rational, whether it expresses our preferences or not (Randall and Downie, 1999). Beauchamp and Childress (2001: 63) explain this belief further by arguing that, 'To respect an autonomous agent is, at a minimum, to acknowledge that person's right to hold views, to make choices, and to take actions based on personal values and beliefs.' Yet simply being human does not automatically give us the right to have our autonomy respected, since there are certain conditions that would also need to be met (Harris, 1985; Gillon, 1985).

- *The first condition of autonomy* is the capacity to reason and make sense of the information imparted (Beauchamp and Childress, 2001). The ability to reason is essential for autonomy; however, there may be varying degrees of autonomy. There are difficulties in formulating a consistently reliable method to determine capacity and decide what capacity entails (Department of Pain Medicine and Palliative Care, 2006). Patients may change their mind, even after choosing a particular treatment. Capacity is therefore not absolute and may vary over time, which highlights a need for constant review. For example, some patients may be unable to understand and retain information, and may not appreciate the consequences of their actions in relation to medication or cancer/progression.
- *The second condition of autonomy* is the ability to clearly express one's own wishes. In relation to terminal sedation this could render a patient incompetent due to their drowsy or unconscious state, which illustrates the dilemmas around using terminal sedation and why this is often considered a last resort at end of life by patients and healthcare professionals.
- *The third condition of autonomy* is the need for decisions to be made free from coercion and controlling influences. However, this may prove difficult since decisions about treatment options in cancer/palliative care are usually made in times of extreme stress/distress. This reflects Sarah's case, where she is pleading for treatment to stay alive for her children.

SHOULD AUTONOMY TAKE PRIORITY OVER OTHER ETHICAL PRINCIPLES?

Autonomy has gained publicity in recent years, partly due to the Mental Capacity Act 2005, which indicated that autonomy should have priority over other ethical principles. While respect for autonomy cannot be absolute (e.g. requests for euthanasia), it raises questions about whether it should override other ethical principles; for example, acute situations where non-consented terminal sedation is required. Within this, terminal sedation may relieve 'suffering'; however, it would also result in the patient permanently being unable to communicate. This raises concerns if the patient's agitation or distress may only have been temporary, since the decision to sedate is rarely revoked.

Similarly, when a patient has specifically requested that analgesia or sedation not be used at the end of life for personal, cultural or religious reasons, this questions whether we should respect their autonomy if their 'suffering' extended to others, or attempt to relieve their suffering using principles of beneficence. Respect for autonomy also requires certain conditions to be met (Harris, 1985; Gillon, 1985). The issue of terminal sedation may be considered a controlling influence with a detrimental effect upon autonomy. This is worrying given the importance of being in control of decisions at the end of life, which is identified as a significant factor in a 'good death' (Smith, 2000).

MILL'S INTERPRETATION OF AUTONOMY

John Stuart Mill claimed that autonomy was important, not because it promoted happiness but because it is a constitutive part of happiness (Gillon, 1985). This is an important point, since if we only believe autonomy to be important because it promotes welfare, then we may have no reason to respect autonomous choices when welfare is not promoted.

Mill also recognised that autonomy could never be absolute, particularly if an autonomous request was deemed harmful to others (Gillon, 1985) – for example, a competent adult's request for euthanasia, since it is unlawful and would place the healthcare professional in an unreasonable position. Respecting another person's autonomy should maximise their overall welfare, since autonomous people are considered to be the best judges of what makes them happy, which reflects a utilitarian view of autonomy. Examples in palliative care may include a competent patient, terminally ill with uncontrolled physical pain who does not want this to be relieved since they want to remain 'in control'. This may reflect their perceptions of a 'good death', rather than another's perception of suffering. To administer analgesia in this situation, without consent, could be considered tantamount to abuse.

Alternatively, a patient's request for terminal sedation may feel unsettling for healthcare professionals, since it may be considered a covert request for euthanasia. However, some patients will openly discuss suicide and request euthanasia to ensure the depth of their suffering has been understood (Coyle et al., 1990, cited in Chater et al., 1998). Therefore, to offer terminal sedation in such situations may be considered a reasonable act. After considering these points, it is clear that Mill and Kant have both contributed to autonomy in medical practice. However, the limitations surrounding autonomy in healthcare must also be considered, particularly if one's actions were to cause harm or deprive others of beneficial acts. This approach highlights Mill's utilitarian beliefs (Mill, 1948).

LIMITATIONS OF RESPECT FOR AUTONOMY

- *The first limitation to autonomy* is that not everyone is autonomous, yet a good death would still matter to those who were not autonomous. Although capacity is included in core ethical principles, a patient's capacity may fluctuate.
- *The second limitation* is whether an autonomous decision should stand if it adversely affects others. Therefore, respect for autonomy can never be absolute.
- *The third limitation* is whether an autonomous choice should always be respected – for example, continuing chemotherapy if it conflicts with beneficence and non-maleficence.

BENEFICENCE

The ethical principle of beneficence refers to a moral obligation to act for the benefit of others by contributing to their overall welfare (Beauchamp and

Childress, 2001). It therefore emphasises the importance of 'doing good to patients' (Hope et al., 2003). As such, acts of beneficence are usually undertaken in terms of mercy, kindness and charity (Beauchamp and Childress, 2001). Beneficence is largely supported by followers of utilitarianism who advocate that the right action would be the one that produces the most happiness (Gillon, 1985). In addition, the philosophers Kant and Ross recognise beneficence as an obligation central to that of deontological ethics (Beauchamp and Childress, 1994). While beneficence may seem central to both morality and humanity, opponents would challenge this fundamental concept on many levels.

First, there are those who argue that we have no real obligation to act beneficently (Beauchamp and Childress, 2001). This position is often referred to as the 'supererogatory' nature of beneficence, which suggests that while beneficence is great, it is above and beyond the call of duty. This viewpoint could therefore lead one to assume that beneficence has more to do with spiritual or religious beliefs.

In fact, some ethical theories, such as certain versions of utilitarianism demand that we always do the act that yields the most good, which clearly would leave no room for such supererogatory acts. Singer, who writes from a strict utilitarian perspective, believes that certain aspects such as third world poverty require us to 'work full time' to bring about relief in doing good, and that in not doing so we would be failing in our moral requirements (McKay, 2002). However, Beauchamp and Childress (2001) suggest that Singer's proposed obligation of beneficence is too demanding since it would require serious disruption in everyday life to benefit those who are sick. Equally, a strict interpretation of Kant's categorical imperative, 'act only on that maxim which one could at the same time will as a universal law' (Gillon, 1985) may also imply that beneficence as a duty is all-pervasive (McKay, 2002).

Yet if we believe that beneficence is supererogatory rather than duty bound, it would be unlikely to supersede that of actual duties. For example, if we have a duty to respect autonomy that conflicts with the demands of beneficence, then duty would always succeed based upon this belief. However, there are those who consider beneficence to be an actual duty, which would mean it would be obligatory to act in a beneficent way. In healthcare there are aspects of obligatory beneficence in action; examples include delivering effective and beneficial treatments for pain or other symptoms and providing sensitive support by assisting patients and families in any way possible. We also know that beneficence and respect for autonomy are two very important ethical principles that lie at the very heart of decision making and which play a vital, integral role in the professional relationship between patients and clinicians.

Certainly, beneficence is the most commonly used principle in the application of care according to the Department of Pain Medicine and Palliative Care (2006). In fact, both nursing and medical professions emphasise the necessity to benefit patients and do no harm through their professional codes of conduct.

Nursing is also strongly influenced by deontology; guidance published by the Nursing and Midwifery Council states that the nurse must 'report [their] concerns in writing if problems in the environment of care are putting people at risk' (NMC, 2008).

The medical profession is primarily guided by the Hippocratic oath, which indicates that physicians should use the treatment available to help the sick, but never with a view to injury and wrongdoing (Faden and Beauchamp, 1986). To follow the principle of beneficence would assume a person's aim is to do what is best for them, given that patients' own ideas are captured by respect for autonomy. Hope et al. (2003) suggest that patients mostly want what is 'objectively in their best interests', yet this presupposes that respecting principles of autonomy and beneficence will arrive at the same conclusion. Indeed, beneficence by definition means 'to do good' which in turn may require 'positive acts' that could contradict a patient's autonomous wishes, believing that 'clinicians know best'; a concept similar to paternalism.

Third, and most importantly, it raises the question of who should judge what is best for an individual patient. This lack of clarity often leads one to assume that beneficence is synonymous with medical paternalism. This point is supported by the fact that clinicians, even after discussion with patients, are not obliged by the prima facie duty of beneficence to do what patients have requested (Gillon, 1985). However, conflict can arise when a competent patient may decide on a course of action clinicians may consider is not in their 'best interests', which reflects Sarah's request to continue 'life-prolonging treatment for cancer'.

Verpoort et al. (2004) attempt to clarify who should judge what is best for individuals by outlining differences between autonomy and beneficence. They suggest that while patient autonomy acknowledges individuals' rights to decide for themselves, beneficence ensures patients' general wellbeing is addressed by 'directed strategies'. However, this explanation only seems to perpetuate the confusion that exists between beneficence and medical paternalism.

MEDICAL PATERNALISM

The distinction between medical paternalism and beneficence is often blurred; Tan (2002) suggests the 'over-emphasis' of beneficence led to the formation of medical paternalism. However, the term 'medical paternalism' conjures up negative images of patients in a subservient position to doctors, where both parties often believe 'the doctor knows best'. Buchanan (1978) suggests that paternalism is the 'interference with a person's liberty of action, where the alleged justification of the interference is that it is for the good of the person whose liberty of action is thus restricted' (Buchanan, 1978: 371).

However, this account suggests underhand tactics through deception, which is immoral and illustrates the immense potential for abuse. Gillon (1985) implies that although deceit in this way still takes place, it can be rationalised as being in the 'patient's best interests'. This clearly illustrates that paternalism has the capacity to be defined and redefined, and is therefore open to interpretation. This suggests there should be increased transparency regarding one's interpretation of paternalism, given advances in medical technology, coupled with ever-increasing publicised cases of negligence.

Dworkin's (1988) philosophical account of paternalism suggests that in order to treat another paternalistically, there must be a violation of their autonomy, which may involve interference with decision making. However, this definition may become less acceptable to the public, given the growing participation in user groups which can directly influence policy and clinical practice.

Conflict may arise in giving chemotherapy to distressed patients who may be incapable of making truly autonomous choices. In such situations some may argue that patients could benefit from doctors making this decision for them, which is often referred to as 'soft paternalism', since patients' autonomy is compromised. In contrast, 'hard paternalism' is where choices are made for others regardless of their level of autonomy (Dworkin, 1988).

If a patient's autonomy is believed to be compromised this may cause concerns for their welfare. However, clinical decisions are still needed, which may require a paternalistic approach. When a patient is believed to have no autonomy, it may be argued that any decision is not paternalistic, which casts doubt on the concept of 'soft paternalism'. Nevertheless, there is clearly a need for paternalism when patients request inappropriate or futile treatments. However, taking Buchanan's (1978) definition of paternalism to its extreme, this suggests that patients need protection from themselves, which increases the premise of 'doctor knows best'. For example, in relation to truth telling, a patient may explicitly request that doctors do not disclose biopsy results if they indicate cancer. This explicit request relies on doctors deciding what is in that patient's best interests; the doctor may decide to give the results outright, regardless of patients' expressed wishes, which reflects definitions of paternalism (Buchanan, 1978; Dworkin, 1988).

In Sarah's case, suddenly imposing bad news when she has specifically asked not to be informed could have catastrophic results if she is not mentally prepared to deal with this. This illustrates that all beneficence is not paternalism, as this act seemed to be motivated by the principle of non-maleficence. While it would also seem that paternalism is motivated by beneficence, this does not mean that you must accept every act done in the name of paternalism. Paternalism appears to be a subset of beneficence, since acts of beneficence can equally be questionable at certain times.

Gillon's (1985) defence of medical paternalism suggests that patients are incapable of making decisions about 'medical problems' as they lack medical knowledge. This presupposes that patients are very unlikely to make the same decisions as doctors, given the implied inequity; there is the assumption that clinicians know more about patients' suffering, which belittles patients' own experiences.

ARGUMENTS IN FAVOUR OF BENEFICENCE OVER AUTONOMY

CASE STUDY 10.1   SARAH (CONTINUED)

Sarah was admitted with symptoms of bowel obstruction during the fifth cycle of palliative chemotherapy and is on parenteral nutrition. Her recent CT scan shows progressive disease, with multiple sites of metastases and bowel obstruction. Sarah did not want to know the results unless they were good, and insists that chemotherapy continues. She refuses to engage in discussions around risks/benefits of treatment and quality of life, future care needs and has declined all community support and hospice referrals.

In relation to Sarah's case, the *first supporting argument* of beneficence is that it offers assistance when decisions are required about treatment and care for non-autonomous patients. This principle is important in cancer and palliative care, when patients are often non-autonomous for long periods of time and may not have made advanced directives, including end of life.

The romanticised view of dying is far removed from reality and can often be less than tranquil. Indeed, there are those who feel that you should not give into death easily, which is echoed in Dylan Thomas's (1951) poem 'Do Not Go Gentle into That Good Night'. However, what alternatives do we have when witnessing over-whelming, possibly intractable distress?

To answer this question, we must remember that the intention of an act is impor-tant since we can never be certain that our actions will have the desired effect, although our premise would be to act beneficently. This may mean not administering terminal sedation as a beneficent act, since this may allow patients to retain aware-ness that their suffering (turmoil and distress) is a sign they are making 'a major adjustment' at the end of life, and not 'going mad' (Stedeford, 1987). Some may conclude that family members and clinicians have a greater duty to support patients in their decision, even if this involves suffering. However, we also have a duty to provide compassionate care and comfort. Ensuring the availability of terminal seda-tion for patients is therefore important, even though it may not be administered.

Austin Cooney (2006) discusses beneficence as resisting the urge to 'do some-thing', which may involve staying alongside patients by validating their emotions. In Sarah's case this focuses around her request not to know bad news, although indicates doubt that all is not well. Equally one's duty to do good may include the realisation that simply 'being with' a patient in times of suffering is not enough, which raises questions of whether it is ever justifiable to withhold sedation using the premise of beneficence? Sarah's case also illustrates that difficult ethical dilem-mas should not be viewed in isolation, which calls for explicit reasoning and clear decision making throughout, together with sensitive, effective communication as a fundamental part of this process.

The second supporting argument of beneficence over respect for autonomy at end of life is the belief that the duty of beneficence lies not with medical staff but with patients themselves. An example would be the need for patients to accept terminal sedation so that the dying process is as peaceful as possible. This would benefit patients by diminishing distress for family members, fellow patients and clinicians, since suffering is not merely confined to patients' own experiences.

Therefore, respecting autonomy does not always override the suffering this may cause to another person. A case in point would be a patient refusing to be in a single side room, which staff feel is necessary to contain psychological distress and/or malodour from a fungating tumour. However, patients may associate moving to a side room with imminent death, and may therefore insist they remain on the main ward. However, this may cause distress for other patients. In this instance, the patient arguably has a duty of beneficence to other patients in the vicinity and also to clinical staff given the problems this may be creating.

Opponents would argue that while terminal sedation may be an acceptable way for clinicians to address intractable symptoms by acting beneficently, we must also be mindful that requests for increasing doses of sedatives may simply be palliating carers' own distress, and this would need to be addressed separately (Kearney, 1996). However, clinicians also have a duty of care to informal caregivers. In respecting patients' wishes, therefore, our actions (or inactions) may inadvertently cause distress to caregivers.

ARGUMENTS AGAINST BENEFICENCE OVER AUTONOMY

The first objection to beneficence is the uncertainty of whether the proposed act produces an overall benefit. In Sarah's case this doubt will be the effect of continuing parenteral nutrition; how can we be sure that continuing it will relieve suffering and become a benevolent act? This creates dilemmas for staff, particularly when there is resistance from family members who may perceive it is 'feeding the cancer' or cessation associated with 'starving her to death'. Doubts regarding which actions are beneficent questions whether our actions are in patients' best interests.

The second objection relates to concerns that palliative sedation may be more beneficial for family/caregivers than individual patients (Austin Cooney, 2006). Lawton's (2000) ethnographic study on patients' experiences of palliative care indicates terminal sedation is not always used beneficently but to promote the ideology of a good death, believing that hospices are 'safe places to suffer'. Janssens et al. (2005) indicate that relatives suffer burnout when patients are sedated for more than two days, suggesting terminal sedation makes dying processes more protracted. Therefore, suggesting that terminal sedation may be a beneficent act appears controversial.

The third objection is that using terminal sedation for patients' benefit makes it difficult for both patients and clinicians to change their mind. If we believe that suffering at end of life is highly dynamic and may offer opportunities for healing (Kearney, 1996), using terminal sedation may prevent the realisation of this potential, since it signifies no way back.

DECISION MAKING

The case study and clinical situations such as terminal sedation highlight experiences of patients, family and clinicians, and different responses. In Sarah's case this may include collusion between staff and family to respect Sarah's wishes. However, hope may change over time and the sanctity of life versus quality of life and dignity can also switch focus over time. While patients can request treatment they cannot demand this, even when the benefit is to be alive. Sarah's case also highlights that some patients do not want to be actively involved in decision making even when competent, which raises issues about what are reasonable expectations, and what clinicians can and should do in such circumstances.

Death may be viewed as a failure by clinicians (Neuberger, 2003). This may create an environment where the culture of care is focused on investigations and invasive procedures, which may be pursued at the expense of comfort care (Ellershaw and Ward, 2003). Equally, patients and their family may be the driving force behind such requests, in their endless search for hope. This may mean that opportunities to prepare patients and their family during the dying process are missed. These are important points to bear in mind, given that most deaths occur in hospital settings (Lawton, 2000). It also highlights the importance of exploring the values, attitudes and beliefs of patients, caregivers and clinicians, which often underpin such discussions.

Decision making in palliative and end of life care should be individualised, including treatment decisions, although this may fluctuate, which calls for constant review with clear communication across professional boundaries and with patients/families. This may include managing conflicting needs and expectations between a patient and their family; in some cases, the family may collude and block discussions to protect their loved one.

COMMUNICATION SKILLS AND DISCLOSING SENSITIVE INFORMATION

Good communication is crucial in oncology and palliative care; determining patients' perceptions, expectations, concerns and needs rely on the communication skills of individual healthcare professionals (Franklin et al., 2015). Good communication skills help to aid understanding of complex information and facilitate decision making. However, the way we communicate with patients can also reduce psychological distress by identifying and assessing their concerns and worries. Although health professionals recognise the importance of this, many patients report a lack of emotional support and communication issues with doctors and nurses (Franklin et al., 2015). During chemotherapy nurses failed to identify

80 per cent of patients' concerns (Farrell et al., 2005), clinicians were often unable to identify patients' preferences and decision-making priorities (Mulley et al., 2012). Identifying and addressing patients' concerns is important, since there are strong correlations between the number and severity of concerns and psychological distress (Harrison et al., 1994; Parle et al., 1996; Farrell et al., 2005). Psychological distress can have a negative impact on decision making since patients can find it hard to understand and assimilate complex information, which can affect their autonomy.

Studies have also demonstrated evidence of blocking behaviours during communication between hospice staff and patients (Heaven and Maguire, 1997; Booth et al., 1996). There may be several reasons for this; however, the strength of patients' emotions and distress may create feelings of anxiety, distress and inadequacy for health professionals. This can make it difficult for clinicians to continue with a challenging interaction and further explore a patient's distress. They will therefore use blocking strategies to avoid further discussions around areas that are painful or threatening to them (Maguire, 1985; Rosenfield and Jones, 2004). However, clinicians may also use blocking strategies to 'protect' the patient, particularly if the person becomes distressed during the consultation, although this can have a negative effect on the patient (Maguire, 1999).

DISCLOSING SENSITIVE INFORMATION

If the news broken does not match what the patient is expecting to hear, this can result in the patient feeling shocked and distressed. It is morally wrong to withhold medical information and deceive patients about their prognosis; clinicians have a duty of care to tailor information to each individual and to exercise sensitivity and compassion when disclosing sensitive information; however, this is often difficult in practice. From a survey of 500 oncologists, 55 per cent reported that 'how to be honest with the patient and not destroy hope' was the most important factor when breaking bad news. However, 39 per cent considered their ability to break bad news was 'fair' while 8 per cent reported this to be 'poor' (Bailea et al., 2000).

SPIKES is a six-step framework for breaking bad news (see Figure 7.1), which enables clinicians to gather information from patients, give medical information, provide support for the patient and develop a plan for the future in collaboration with the patient (Bailea et al., 2000). However, before giving any information it is crucial to gather information from patients about their perceptions and expectations, their knowledge and understanding, and any concerns or worries they may have. If this is not achieved the clinician will not have a full understanding of what the patient knows, what they understand, and how they feel, including their concerns. Exploring this initially is a good investment of time for clinicians, since it will make it easier to facilitate communication and shared decision making.

This strategy fits with 'breaking bad news' and processes for giving complex information; it should not be rushed and aims to provide clear and open communication delivered with compassion. It is also considered good practice to have a have a family member present when significant news is imparted, which appears to be what Sarah was requesting. Sarah's case also highlights the importance of checking a patient's perceptions, particularly when ordering investigations such as a CT scan, since this may have implications for symptoms experienced and perceptions regarding their significance in relation to the cancer, and how further imaging may relate to a patient's goals of care and future treatment. Chapter 7 discusses the medical perspective on breaking bad news using the SPIKES model.

HOW DO WE ENSURE THAT WE ARE BEING ETHICAL IN OUR DAY-TO-DAY PRACTICE?

The benefits of teamworking in hospital contexts are well known, in particular for creating opportunities to allow for more considered decision making. Teamworking actively encourages ethical discussions to be made as a group. It can also help avoid 'compassion fatigue' and 'moral burnout', which should not be underestimated, coupled with the ongoing importance of early integration of supportive and palliative care, rather than palliative care being considered as an 'add on' after active treatment has 'failed', with frantic discussions when people are dying.

Clinicians should also be mindful of the professional language they use when discussing sensitive issues at the end of life such as 'futility', which can be viewed by the public as 'they can't be bothered' or may convey something 'bad'. Also, the phrases 'save life and prevent death' require further exploration in day-to-day practice.

In healthcare, difficult decisions are being made daily, including moral questions around 'life at all costs', resource allocation, 'false hope versus no hope' and 'dealing with uncertainty'. In balancing hope versus telling the truth, some of the key ethical dilemmas and questions clinicians often ask within palliative care include:

- How can we sustain life?
- Should we sustain life?
- Is there any ethical difference between withholding and withdrawing life-prolonging treatment?
- Is withholding and withdrawing life-prolonging treatment tantamount to euthanasia?

DO NOT ATTEMPT RESUSCITATION ORDERS (DNAR)

The case of Tracey v Cambridge University Hospital (EWCA, 2014; RCUK, 2014a) raised some important points about the documentation of DNAR instructions in patients' notes, communication with patients and their families, and respect for patients' autonomy. In a statement by the UK Research Council it said, 'This case highlights a highly complex area of medical practice and ethics' (RCUK, 2014b).

The judgment from the Court of Appeal stated that the hospital was in breach of Tracey's human rights (Article 8 of the European Convention) by failing to discuss DNAR with her when she had capacity and wanted to be involved in decisions about her care (RCUK, 2014b). An article by the solicitors in this case provides a clear summary of the key points and implications (Evans, 2014).

The case highlights some of the difficulties with open discussions, which may create fear amongst medical staff about discussing potential medical treatment when there is no, or limited, prospect of recovery/benefit. Similarly, open discussions about cardiopulmonary resuscitation (CPR) can be challenging, particularly if the patient's family perceive that it is likely to be effective and thus demand it as a medical intervention. Some important questions for health professionals to consider in relation to treatment decision making and care planning in the last 12 months of life include:

- Has the patient got capacity?
- Is there an advanced directive to refuse treatment?
- Is there an advance care plan?
- Is there an escalation of care/ceilings of care discussion?
- What are the benefits, risks and implications?
- Who should be involved?

CONCLUSION

This chapter has discussed the main ethical approaches of consequentialism and deontology to explore the key ethical principles within palliative care: respect for autonomy, beneficence, justice and paternalism. They are discussed within the context of professional codes of conduct and current NHS guidelines and resources, using a case study to highlight key points within clinical practice and areas for reflection. Addressing aspects that constitute a benevolent act has raised important issues around who should judge what is best for individual patients and implications for medical paternalism.

The chapter has provided an ongoing debate about respect for autonomy and beneficence in order to highlight dilemmas in daily clinical practice in palliative care for patients, caregivers and clinicians, and how these may be addressed. Supporting arguments of beneficence over respecting autonomy may be in direct opposition to patients' or clinicians' own beliefs and values at end of life, including ideals of achieving 'a good death'. Within this, the intention of the act is all-important, given the lack of certainty that our actions will have the desired effect, the complexities within palliative care/end of life, and individual variability. The objections offered against beneficence over autonomy include the need to demonstrate that an act is truly beneficent, even where it is considered to be in the patient's best interest. Without absolute certainty, we cannot profess that an action is wholly beneficent.

REFERENCES

Austin Cooney, G. (2006) *Palliative Sedation: The Ethical Controversy*. www.medscape.com/viewarticle (11 September 2006), pp.1–5.

Bailea, W.F., Buckman, R., Lenzia, R., Globera, G., Bealea, E.A. and Kudelkab, A.P. (2000) 'SPIKES – a six-step protocol for delivering bad news: application to the patient with cancer.' *The Oncologist*, 5 (4): 302–11.

Baracos, V.E. (2013) 'Clinical trials of cancer cachexia therapy, now and hereafter.' *AmJ Clin Oncol*, 31(10): 1257–8. doi: 10.1200/JCO.2012.48.3149

Beauchamp, T.L. and Childress, J.F. (2001) *Principles of Biomedical Ethics*. 5th ed. New York: Oxford University Press.

Booth, K., Maguire, P., Butterworth, T., Hillier, V. (1996) 'Perceived professional support and the use of blocking behaviours by hospice nurses'. *Journal of Advanced Nursing*, 24: 522–27.

Bozzetti, F., Arends, J., Lundholm, K., Micklewright, A., Zurcher, G., Muscaritoli, M. (2009) 'ESPEN Guidelines on Parenteral Nutrition: non-surgical oncology.' *Clin Nutr*, 28(4): 445–54. doi: 10.1016/j.clnu.2009.04.011

Buchanan, A. (1978) 'Medical paternalism.' *Philosophy and Public Affairs*, 7(4): 370–90.

Buckman, R. (1992) *Breaking Bad News: A Guide for Health Care Professionals*. Baltimore. Johns Hopkins University Press. p15.

Chater, S., Viola, R., Paterson, J. and Jarvis, V. (1998) 'Sedation for intractable distress in the dying: a survey of experts.' *Palliative Medicine*, 12: 255–69.

Department of Pain Medicine and Palliative Care (2006) *Ethics and Legal Issues in Palliative Care*. Available at www.wehealny.org/stoppain/palliative_careold/ethics.html

Dworkin, G. (1988) *Theory and Practice of Autonomy*. Cambridge: Cambridge University Press.

Ellershaw, J. and Ward, C. (2003) 'Care of the dying patient: the last hours or days of life.' *BMJ*, 326: 30–3.

England and Wales Court of Appeal (2014) Decisions. *EWCA Civ 822*. www.bailii.org/cgi-bin/markup.cgi?doc=/ew/cases/EWCA/Civ/2014/822.html&query=Tracey+and+v+and+Cambridge&method=boolean#disp32, accessed November 2017.

Evans, S. (2014) *An Issue of Life or Death* ... Available at www.hempsons.co.uk/news-articles/issue-life-death, accessed November 2017.

Faden, R.R. and Beauchamp T.L. (1986) *A History and Theory of Informed Consent*. Oxford: Oxford University Press.

Farrell, C., Heaven, C., Beaver, K. and Maguire, P. (2005) 'Identifying the concerns of women undergoing chemotherapy.' *Patient Education and Counselling*, 56 (1): 72–7.

Faull, C. and Blankley, L. (2015) *Palliative Care*. 2nd ed. Oxford: Oxford University Press.

Frankin, A., Green, C. and Schofield, N. (2015) 'Compassionate and effective communication: key skills and principles', in C. Farrell (ed.), *Advanced Nursing Practice and Nurse-Led Clinics in Oncology*. London: Routledge.

General Medical Council (2010) *Treatment and Care towards the End of Life: Good Practice in Decision Making*. Available at http://tinyurl.com/lgrq7qn, accessed 4 June 2014.

Gillon, R. (1985) *Philosophical Medical Ethics*. Chichester: Wiley.

Good, P., Richard, R., Syrmis, W., Jenkins-Marsh, S. and Stephens, J. (2014) 'Medically assisted nutrition to assist palliative care patients.' *The Cochrane Database of Systematic Reviews*. doi: 10.1002/14651858.CD006274.pub3

Hagerty, R.G., Butow, P.N., Ellis, P.M., Lobb, E.A., et al. (2005) 'Communicating with realism and hope: incurable cancer patients' views on the disclosure of prognosis.' *Journal of Clinical Oncology*, 23 (6): 1278–88.

Harris, J. (1985) *The Value of Life*. London: Routledge.

Harrison, J., Maguire, P., Ibbotson, T., Macleod, R. and Hopwood, P. (1994) 'Concerns, confiding and psychiatric disorders in newly diagnosed cancer patients: a descriptive study.' *Psycho-Oncology, 3* (3): 173–9.

Heaven, C. and Maguire, P. (1997) 'Disclosure of concerns by hospice patients and their identification by nurses.' *Palliative Medicine, 11* (4): 283–90.

Hope, T., Savulescu, J. and Hendrick, J. (2003) *Medical Ethics and Law. The Core Curriculum.* Edinburgh: Elsevier Science.

Janssens, R., Olthuis, G. and Dekkers, W. (2005) 'Terminal sedation and dehydration go hand in hand.' *International Journal of Palliative Nursing, 11* (7): 334–5.

Kearney, M. (1996) *Mortally Wounded.* Dublin: Marino Books.

Lawton, J. (2000) *The Dying Process: Patients' Experiences of Palliative Care.* London: Routledge.

Maguire, P. (1985) 'Barriers to psychological care of the dying.' *BMJ, 291* (6510): 1711–13.

Maguire, P. (1999) 'Improving communication with cancer patients.' *European Journal of Cancer, 35* (10): 1415–22.

McKay, A.C. (2002) 'Supererogation and the profession of medicine.' *Journal of Medical Ethics, 28*: 70–3.

Mental Capacity Act 2005, Chapter 9.

Mill, J.S. (1948) *On Liberty.* London: George Routledge and Sons.

Mulley, A., Trimble, C. and Elwyn, G. (2012) *Patients' Preferences Matter: Stop the Silent Misdiagnosis.* London: The King's Fund.

National Cancer Institute (2013) *Nutrition in Cancer Care: Nutrition in Advanced Cancer.* Available at http://tinyurl.com/8xfdwvr, accessed 29 October 2013.

National Confidential Enquiry into Patient Outcome and Deaths (NCEPOD) (2008) *Systemic Anti-Cancer Therapy: For Better, for Worse.* Available at www.ncepod.org.uk/2008sact.html, accessed 4 June 2018.

Neuberger, J. (2003) 'Commentary: a "good death" is possible in the NHS.' *BMJ, 326*: 34.

Nursing and Midwifery Council (NMC) (2008) *The Code: Standards of Conduct, Performance and Ethics for Nurses and Midwives.* London: NMC.

O'Neill, O. (2002) *Autonomy and Trust in Bioethics.* Cambridge: Cambridge University Press.

Oxford English Dictionary (2017) Definition of 'ethics'. Available at https://en.oxforddiction aries.com/definition/ethics, accessed November 2017.

Parle, M., Jones, B. and Maguire, P. (1996) 'Maladaptive coping and affective disorders in cancer patients.' *Psychological Medicine, 26*: 735–44.

Randall, F. and Downie, R.S. (1999) *Palliative Care Ethics. A Companion for All Specialties.* 2nd ed. Oxford: Oxford Medical Press.

Resuscitation Council (UK) (RCUK) (2014a) *Statements.* Available at www.resus.org.uk/statements/tracey-v-cuh-and-secretary-of-state-for-health, accessed November 2017.

Resuscitation Council (UK) (RCUK) (2014b) *Tracey Judgement Statement.* Available at file:///C:/Users/Carole/Downloads/Tracey_judgement_Statement.pdf, accessed November 2017.

Rosenfield, P.J. and Jones, L. (2004) 'Striking a balance: training medical students to provide empathetic care.' *Medical Education, 38* (9): 927–33.

Royal College of Physicians (2010) *Oral Feeding Difficulties and Dilemmas: A Guide to Practical Care, Particularly towards the End of Life. Report of a Working Party.* Available at http://tinyurl.com/m453vmr, accessed 4 June 2014.

Smith, R. (2000) 'A good death.' *BMJ, 320*: 129–30.

Stedeford, A. (1987) 'Hospice: a safe place to suffer?' *Palliative Medicine, 1*: 73–4.

Tan, N.H.S.S. (2002) 'Deconstructing paternalism – what serves the patient best?' *Singapore Medical Journal, 43* (3): 148–51.

Thomas, D. (1951) 'Do Not Go Gentle into That Good Night'. Available at www.bbc.co.uk/wales/dylanthomas/bibliography (14/10/2006).

Tracey v C UH and Secretary of State for health-resuscitation council. Available at www.resus.org.uk/statements/tracey-v-cuh-and-secretary-of-state-for-health

Verpoort, C., Gastmans, C., De Bal, N. and Dierckx de Casterlé, B. (2004) 'Nurses' attitudes to euthanasia: A review of the literature.' *Nursing Ethics*, *11*, 349–65.

FURTHER READING

Jackson, S. and Vernon, M. (1998)'Respecting patients' autonomy-a case report'. *Journal of Nursing Care*, Spring, pp.11–12.

Jeffrey, D. (1993)'Autonomy in palliative care' *Managing Cancer*, Glaxo Labs Ltd., 2 (2): 4–6.

11

HOSPITAL PALLIATIVE CARE TEAMS

ANNE-MARIE RAFTERY

LEARNING OUTCOMES

- Describe the role of the hospital palliative care teams
- Describe how referral to palliative care teams in hospitals assists integration between palliative care specialists and nurses
- Identify the importance of shared decision making when exploring the patient's/family's/ clinician's goals and values
- Discuss advance care planning (ACP) with patients and families and their role in increasing the knowledge and confidence of both generalist and specialist clinicians

INTRODUCTION

This chapter highlights the key features of the patient's journey in hospital, from diagnosis through to end of life. It begins by explaining the role of the specialist palliative care clinicians, often referred to as the hospital palliative care team (HPCT) or supportive care team.

The chapter will briefly trace the origins of and establishment of such teams and their role in influencing the care, treatment and education of patients and healthcare professionals. It will also consider the composition of the HPCT and the role of the clinical nurse specialist in the referral of patients, links with other members of the multidisciplinary team (MDT) and their liaison role across hospital and community.

In particular, the chapter focuses on how symptom management can be influenced by the involvement of such teams working in conjunction with hospital staff, which evidence suggests underutilise this valuable resource. Collaboration with clinicians to embed and incorporate early supportive and palliative care is therefore crucial through joint working and in close partnership.

ORIGINS AND ESTABLISHMENT OF HOSPITAL PALLIATIVE CARE TEAMS

There are many terms associated with palliative care which, although inter-related, help frame and explain the introduction and concept of hospital palliative care teams (HPCT) and how they have evolved over the years, particularly in the UK.

This plethora of terms, ranging from 'palliative care', 'end of life care', 'supportive care', 'best supportive care', 'terminal care' and 'hospice care' although used interchangeably assumes an agreed meaning amongst healthcare professionals, patients, carers and members of the public alike. Yet there is often inconsistency in how these terms are interpreted, applied and even defined in both palliative/oncology literature and national/public documents. As a necessary first step, it therefore seems important to outline these common terms in relation to the specific similarities and differences with each approach in this context.

COMMON TERMS

PALLIATIVE CARE

Palliative care as defined by the World Health Organization (1990) is an approach that aims to improve the quality of life of patients and their families who are living with a life-threatening illness. It is achieved through the prevention and relief of suffering, early identification and relief of pain and other distressing symptoms, using a holistic approach focusing on physical, psychosocial and spiritual aspects. This both affirms life and considers dying as a normal process.

It is now widely accepted that palliative care is often appropriate much earlier in the course of a life-threatening illness and should not merely be reserved for patients with a cancer diagnosis or those who are imminently dying (National Council for Hospice and Specialist Palliative Care Services, 2002; National Institute for Health Care Excellence, 2004; Department of Health (DoH), 2008; National Palliative and End of Life Care Partnership, 2015).

Yet, despite this knowledge, palliative care is still interpreted amongst some oncology healthcare professionals as being synonymous with terminal care (Bruera and Hui, 2012), which has resulted in some HPCTs, particularly in the UK and USA, 'rebranding' or changing their name from palliative care to supportive care, given they feel the name 'palliative care' can pose a real barrier for healthcare professionals and patients/carers alike in accessing this vital service.

SUPPORTIVE CARE

The term supportive care has been in existence for some time (DoH, 2008; National Institute for Health and Clinical Excellence (NICE), 2004), and is defined by the Multinational Association of Supportive Care in Cancer (MASCC, 2013) as the prevention and management of the adverse side effects of cancer and its treatment, from diagnosis through to end of life care, encompassing the alleviation of symptoms and the complications of cancer, while easing the emotional burden of patients and caregivers. NICE (2004) also suggests that supportive care is an umbrella term for all services that may be required, based on an assumption of needs from diagnosis onwards. Palliative care is thus an important part of supportive care and embraces many elements indicated by NICE (2004).

It could be argued that supportive care is merely a pseudonym for palliative care and that supportive care and palliative care are in fact one and the same, perhaps with a stronger emphasis in relation to supportive care – supporting patients undergoing anti-cancer therapies in the last year of life. Currently the term supportive care does not appear to have any negative connotations with death and dying. Yet some palliative care professionals consider this to be only a matter of time, and that changing the name from palliative to supportive care merely avoids the heart of the matter by creating a lack of transparency and honesty in what is being offered.

BEST SUPPORTIVE CARE

While 'supportive care' and 'best supportive care' are phrases that arguably sound the same and are often used interchangeably, they actually represent different key points in the patient's cancer trajectory. In fact, 'best supportive care' is interpreted by generalist health professionals as indicating no further active treatment interventions are either appropriate or offered, which is often viewed as a prerequisite to terminal care. However, it is not clear whether the term is directly discussed with patients or carers when a referral is made to supportive/palliative care teams in both hospital and community settings.

END OF LIFE CARE

In the last decade, the term 'end of life care' emerged in both cancer and non-malignancy, perhaps reinforced by the National End of Life Care Strategy (DoH, 2008) relating to the vision for services across the UK.

However, the definition of end of life care is currently being debated in the UK in response to criticisms around the Liverpool Care Pathway for the Dying Patient (LCP) following The Independent Review of the Liverpool Care Pathway (2013). The fact that end of life care can mean any period between the last year of life of a person with a chronic and progressive disease to the last hours or days of life is clearly open to misinterpretation given this diverse continuum.

It is clear then that end of life care encompasses both supportive and palliative care, focusing care not only as the person is in the final hours or days of life, but, more broadly, on the care of all people with a terminal illness that has become advanced.

In fact, 'end of life' appears to be a term used more and more frequently in the UK by both healthcare professionals and the public to describe a person who is entering the last few weeks and days of life, rather than the last year of life. This can result in misinterpretation, unless healthcare professionals are clear about the meaning of terms used and the care being delivered, to avoid unnecessary distress to patients and their families, which arose following the controversy in the media in 2013 around the LCP. For the purpose of clarity within this chapter, end of life care is interpreted as representing the last year of someone's life.

TERMINAL CARE AND HOSPICE CARE

Terminal care has been synonymous with hospice care, which began in the UK in the mid 1960s by Dame Cicely Saunders, founder of the modern hospice movement. She emphasised the importance of viewing patients holistically, yet had the foresight to recommend palliative care be incorporated into modern medicine. Her statement that 'You matter because you are you and you matter to the end of your life. We will do all we can not only to help you die peacefully, but also to live until you die' eloquently encapsulates her overall aim. This may also explain the evolvement of hospital palliative care teams and the growing trend of the palliative care approach in non-malignant disease, perhaps fuelled by a need to ensure equity of access across a range of settings and all life-limiting conditions. Hospice care in the UK can be accessed for any patient with a life-limiting illness (not just cancer) at any point across the illness continuum. Hospices often provide care in a day case setting, outpatient clinic or admission for respite, symptom control or terminal care with ongoing bereavement support. Most are supported by charities, although some receive a proportion of funding from the National Health Service.

Due to their heavy reliance on general public support through fundraising, this has forced hospices to examine the way they have traditionally provided palliative care services. Until recently, this has predominantly been for patients with a cancer diagnosis, which led to many hospices rebranding in order to update their image and reconfigure their services to include provision for any patient with a life-limiting illness.

HOSPITAL PALLIATIVE CARE TEAMS

Palliative care, with its origins in the hospice movement, was thus considered the gold standard. However, with the majority of people dying in hospital (Royal College of Physicians, 2016; National Palliative and End of Life Care Partnership, 2015), there was a need to improve the quality of care and standards, and hospital-based palliative care teams were an ideal way of doing this. In general, specialist palliative care professionals working in district general hospitals or cancer centres aim to work alongside an oncology or primary care team without directly taking over the patient's care, with the exception of inpatient hospice settings. In fact, some HPCTs have become 'integrated teams', which means they are one team working across hospital and community settings, with no clear demarcation, with the aim of improving continuity and ultimately the 'patient experience'.

Hospital palliative care teams network closely with colleagues across hospital, community and hospice settings and are seen as an invaluable resource, particularly in difficult and distressing situations and those where considerable ongoing support to a patient and family is required, as often even broaching end of life conversations can be very difficult, as the words uttered can often confirm both the patient's and healthcare professionals' own fears about mortality.

An important distinction across primary and secondary care settings is that palliative care can, and should be, delivered by generalists and specialists alike. Certainly in the UK, palliative care is no longer merely associated with cancer, but any life-limiting illness such as dementia or end stage renal or heart disease. In fact, more recently, patients admitted to some hospitals considered 'elderly and frail' were automatically being referred to HPCT services on this basis, given the assumption they would undoubtedly have palliative care needs. Yet this knee jerk reaction to refer *all* patients in this client group may result in future demand outweighing capacity, leaving supportive/palliative care teams overstretched and at risk of burnout.

It seems worth drawing distinctions between generic and specialist palliative care, since palliative care/supportive care teams are unable to, and do not necessarily need to, see every patient with palliative care needs. In fact, one of the main aims of palliative care as a philosophy is not to deskill the generalist workforce but further enhance their skills, knowledge and confidence through education and training and specialist support (Skilbeck and Payne, 2005). Seeing all patients with non-specialist palliative care needs would thus result in a deskilled workforce.

Generic palliative care can be viewed as an adoption of the palliative care approach by the workforce, which focuses on quality of life using a whole-person or holistic approach. Within this are essential central components that encompass the person and those that matter to them, including respect for autonomy/choice and emphasis on open and honest communication.

Specialist palliative care primarily focuses on management of complex pain, symptom control and psychological distress for patients and carers from diagnosis onwards, including supportive, palliative care in the last days of life. Key points of referral to community or HPCT would include complex symptom management and psychosocial support.

TEAM STRUCTURE

The palliative care team is often based in hospital but exists in the community, usually comprising a consultant or consultants in palliative medicine and clinical nurse specialists in palliative care. Other team members may also make a significant contribution to the team in a part- or full-time capacity or be called upon as and when needed as extended members of the specialist palliative care MDT. Commonly, teams can consist of chaplaincy, bereavement support, dieticians, physical and occupational therapists, discharge planning nurses, complementary therapy staff, counsellors and social workers. This team would usually meet on a weekly basis to discuss ongoing patients and those newly referred who require a multiprofessional team approach to supportive/palliative care delivery.

MACMILLAN NURSES

In the UK, some clinical nurse specialists in palliative care are called Macmillan nurses, whether working in hospital or community, providing support and advice from diagnosis onwards. The Macmillan title represents initial funding from the Macmillan charity for the postholder's salary, and may also apply to other healthcare professionals such as consultants in palliative medicine and allied health professionals. However, Macmillan nurses are often associated by the public as synonymous with terminal care, an image that the Macmillan charity is working hard to correct.

However, as a Macmillan clinical nurse specialist in palliative care working in a cancer centre, the hospital supportive care team I work with would become involved at any point in the patient's 'cancer journey'. This spectrum may include from diagnosis, such as management of mucositis following radical radiotherapy for head and neck cancer; refractory nausea/vomiting following stem cell transplantation; physical symptoms associated with malignant bowel obstruction in advanced ovarian cancer, including psychological support and ethical decision making around artificial nutrition while receiving chemotherapy with palliative intent. At the other end of the spectrum it might include terminal care, where a patient may have been admitted for symptom control while receiving anti-cancer therapy but suddenly deteriorates acutely and dies in the cancer centre, which the patient may have requested as their preferred place of care and/or death.

This model is slightly different from most hospital palliative care teams in that the HPCT purely see patients with a cancer diagnosis given it is a cancer centre and often see the most difficult and complex of cases, including a younger population.

With this in mind, the role of the HPCT within the cancer centre is to meet the supportive, palliative and end of life care needs of patients and their carer(s) from diagnosis onwards, including treatment-related problems using an MDT approach. Thus the team provides an all-inclusive 'enhanced supportive care in cancer model' which incorporates closer working between the services that support cancer patients and more integrated working with oncology teams, with earlier involvement in patient care.

The aim is to:

- facilitate an integrated MDT approach to address the physical, psychological, spiritual and social concerns of patients and their carer(s)
- enable timely liaisons across primary, secondary, social and voluntary sector care to enable continuity of care and increased patient choice
- support and guide specialist staff in the care of patients with complex supportive, palliative and end of life care needs
- develop education, audit and research activities relating to supportive, palliative and end of life care across the cancer centre and cancer network

REFERRALS TO HOSPITAL PALLIATIVE CARE TEAMS

There are different HPCT models that can differ widely across the UK. As there are no nationally agreed referral criteria, the common themes appear to be *complexity*, due in part to patient need and the *confidence/skill of the non-specialist clinician* or workforce. However, the HPCT I work with would see patients and their carer(s) with specialist palliative care needs from diagnosis onwards, right through to end of life.

Referrals can be from any ward or outpatient service and relate to:

- difficult complex pain and symptoms
- advice and management of treatment-related symptoms
- psychosocial support for patient/carer(s)
- complex end of life care/future planning
- rapid discharge for care in the last few weeks/days of life

Referrals to the HPCT are agreed with the patient's own medical team, the only exception being a self-referral from a patient/carer which is sent to the HPCT indicating the patient's details, reasons for referral including any medication the patient may be taking and the level of urgency of the referral. Table 11.1 provides an overview of all the possible reasons for HPCT referral. The HPCT aims to review a patient within 24 hours of a referral being received. Contact will be maintained with the patient/carer and clinical team(s) until the symptoms/concerns have stabilised and there is either no need for specialist supportive care, the patient no longer wishes to access the service or the needs of the patient can be met by the hospital-based clinical teams or primary care services.

The HPCT also triage referrals from outpatient/day case areas through a designated bleep, which is held by one of the clinical nurse specialists with calls triaged according to the level of complexity and urgency – for example, verbal advice, immediate review and/or referral into the weekly pain and symptom control clinic. Furthermore, oncology teams are encouraged to notify the HPCT of a forthcoming appointment where a joint review is required. Table 11.1 provides an illustration of some of the common reasons for referral to the HPCT.

Table 11.1   Common reasons for referral to HPCT

PHYSICAL	PSYCHOLOGICAL
• Pain – bone, visceral, neuropathic • Nausea/vomiting • Ascites • Constipation • Dyspnoea • Pruritus • Hiccups • Anorexia • Fatigue • Sweating • Seizures • Fungating wounds • Terminal agitation • Respiratory tract secretions • Haemorrhage	• Anxiety and adjustment disorder • Depression • Total pain/distress • Confusion • Agitation • Patient and family distress • Staff support • End of treatment discussions • Transition of care to end of life/palliative/ terminal care
SOCIAL	SPIRITUAL
• Complex discharge planning • Hospice care • Bereavement support	• Faith practices, beliefs and rituals • Spiritual anguish • Suffering • Terminal care • Terminal agitation • Family/carer distress
COMMUNICATION ISSUES	ETHICAL ISSUES
• Dealing with significant news • Managing conflict • Goals of care • Advance care planning	• Artificial nutrition • Resuscitation • Support in weighing up risks/burdens vs. benefits of treatments

SUPPORTIVE/PALLIATIVE CARE CLINICS

Additional specialist supportive and palliative care advice can also be sought through a weekly supportive/palliative care clinic. The clinic is run by palliative medicine consultants, consultant in pain management, nurse specialists, pharmacy and complementary therapy. This integrated approach enables joint reviews and discussion and thus provides a coordinated and holistic approach. Written referrals are received from both oncology teams within the cancer centre and primary care – for example, GP and community Macmillan teams. The HPCT again would maintain contact until the symptoms/concerns had stabilised.

SEVEN-DAY SUPPORTIVE/PALLIATIVE CARE

Most HPCTs in the UK also provide a seven-day face-to face service during the working hours of the working week, usually provided by nurse specialists with telephone access to senior palliative care advice/support available if required.

Telephone advice outside of these times may also be available via the local hospice 24-hour telephone advice services.

There are challenges working in cancer and specialist palliative care, not least difficulties with diagnosing the dying phase. This is due in part to the complexity and acuity of patients undergoing complex treatments which may continue right up until several months before their death, coupled with clinicians not wanting to take away hope, which can result in honest and realistic conversations not taking place. In addition, there are concerns that a framework such as the LCP no longer exists, which non-specialists felt was a really useful aid memoire to providing good care in the last days of life.

COLLABORATING AND INFLUENCING CARE

The landscape of cancer is changing, with sophisticated screening and targeted/improved treatments resulting in more people living longer, with some cancers, such as certain types of breast cancer, now viewed as a chronic disease.

Yet we know that certain cancers such as haemopoietic cancers historically under-utilise supportive/palliative care resources and could benefit from early integration of palliative care for patients and their families (Marie Curie, 2016). The goal of supportive/palliative care is to improve care, particularly for those patients at high risk of complex symptom clusters, non-relapse mortality or relapse. This would offer an opportunity to clarify goals of care, advance care planning and improve the quality of care for both recipients and families. The reasons for delayed referral to supportive/palliative care in haemopoietic cancers are well documented and multifaceted, and may include feelings of failure by the clinician in some cases of giving up or losing hope, particularly when a patient they may have known for many years has progressed (Manitta et al., 2010).

There is also mounting evidence from the USA (Temel et al., 2010) in relation to the benefit of early palliative care in cancer care linked with improved survival and quality of life, optimisation of timing of chemotherapy, reduced need for aggressive treatments at end of life and improved care in the last days of life with lower overall healthcare costs.

This proactive rather than reactive approach has certainly influenced the care delivered at the cancer centre in the north-west of England, which pioneered the model of 'enhanced supportive care in cancer'. This approach is essentially about collaborative working with clinicians to promote early palliative care integration. The importance of working together across disciplines and settings cannot be underestimated with benefits which include:

* support in decision making
* exploring the patient's and clinician's goals and values when making treatment-based decisions
* exploring the decision-making process
* introducing advance care planning

Up-skilling generalists through joint working and collaboration not only improves their knowledge of symptom management and increases their confidence in communication skills, but also improves the HPCT's knowledge first-hand in disease-specific treatments, with oncologists more likely to refer to the HPCT in the future.

Improving Supportive and Palliative Care in Adults with Cancer (NICE, 2004) clearly recognised palliative care as a key point in the patient pathway following diagnosis, which may be offered at the same time as active treatments. In fact, palliative care is now considered as having equal weighting in terms of essential services alongside surgery, radiotherapy and chemotherapy – in essence the '4th pillar of cancer care' (NHS England, 2016).

However, one cannot help but wonder what the future holds after adopting such a proactive approach in supportive/palliative care. We know the tide is beginning to turn with earlier palliative care involvement, which has historically been at the latter stages of the disease trajectory. Yet the question is whether as a profession, supportive/palliative care is fit for the future given the challenges and opportunities that lie ahead, and whether generalists and specialists can realistically deal with the sheer number of patients likely to be referred using this proactive approach.

An ageing population, increasing comorbidity and improvements in healthcare brings increasing expectations of high-quality supportive, palliative and end of life care, with palliative care quite rightly now seen as a basic human right. Many healthcare professionals argue this will 'open the floodgates to all non-malignant disease'. As a profession, supportive/palliative care must therefore look to the future and ensure its members are resilient to this changing landscape (Goodrich et al., 2015) in order to reduce the risk of stress and burnout within the profession, and remain specialists in their own right. Otherwise the phrases 'be careful what you wish for' and 'Jack of all trades, master of none' immediately spring to mind.

Another concern is that in trying to see patients far earlier in the cancer journey, including patients living with and beyond cancer, one wonders whether palliative care clinicians indeed have the skill set and knowledge to manage this growing cohort of patients. It could be argued that perhaps the biggest lesson from the downfall of the Liverpool Care Pathway was the assumption that the complexities around dying were fully embedded and taken on by generalists.

One way of avoiding overburdening the supportive/palliative care system is through a standardised referral pathway, for example using a screening tool such as the Palliative Care Outcome Scale (POS). The POS measures are specifically developed for use with people with advanced diseases (e.g. cancer) and non-malignant disease (e.g. respiratory, heart, renal or liver failure and neurological diseases). The POS measures palliative care needs rather than prognostication and can also be used in audit, research and training which has been used successfully across Europe, Australia, Asia, Africa and America. With the advent of newer targeted treatments, timely discussions such as advance care planning in end of life care may often be left until the last few months/weeks of life for similar reasons.

ADVANCE CARE PLANNING

Advance care planning (ACP) is an important part of optimal palliative care and has been discussed in earlier chapters, most notably Chapter 3 in relation to patients with advanced dementia. ACP is best described as a process of ongoing discussion which can be both informal and formal between an individual/patient, their family and healthcare professional(s) in anticipation of deterioration and end of life care. ACP is a prediction of needs, not prognostication. It allows care preferences to be understood and documented, including treatment, symptom control and goals of care and may include advanced wishes such as preferred place of care and death, or the appointment of a decision maker before the patient loses capacity. Exploration of these topics allows the patient to discover what is important to them and empowers patients to have a say about their current and future care (Krishnan et al., 2017).

Advance care planning identifies patients who may be entering the last year of life and aims to assess their current and future care and personal needs while planning across boundaries.

The benefits of ACP include increased patient and family satisfaction, reduced stress and a reduction in psychological morbidity in surviving relatives (Detering et al., 2010). Yet most patients want the clinician to start the discussion and thus wait for the discussion to happen, while most clinicians wait for patients to raise the topic, which results in conversations around ACP rarely taking place (Momen and Barclay, 2011).

Advance care planning discussions therefore require the patient to have a good understanding of their current and future health/treatment and care options, and the benefits and consequences of any decision. It requires the healthcare professional to have the skills to assess a patient's perceptions and concerns, potentially confirm or deliver distressing information and to handle strong emotions. The clinical nurse specialist thus has an important role in holistic assessments including physical, psychological, social and spiritual aspects, linking with other key members of the multidisciplinary team. This also includes liaison with family members in the community and requires an ability to foster good working relationships across all clinical settings, together with excellent communication skills, including negotiating skills and managing conflict, since goals of care may differ within professions and/or between the patient and their family.

CONCLUSION

This chapter has described the composition of hospital palliative care teams, their importance in providing optimal palliative care for patients and their supportive role in enabling families to come to terms with end of life care. The team is also a resource available to hospital clinicians who may be considered generalists in relation to palliative care. The chapter has stressed the importance of collaborative working between specialists and generalists in order to promote early palliative care referral and integration. By communicating directly with the hospital team, clinicians can and do receive valuable assistance in the complex and often sensitive issue of shared decision making, which involves exploring the patient's and clinician's goals and values when making treatment-based decisions. Moreover, like other chapters in the book, this chapter has discussed advance care planning and the importance of this being conducted informally and formally in a timely fashion, while increasing the knowledge and confidence of both generalist and specialist clinicians.

REFERENCES

Bruera, E. and Hui, D. (2012) 'Conceptual models for integrating palliative care at cancer centres.' *Journal of Palliative Medicine, 15* (11): 1261–9.

Department of Health (2008) *End of Life Care Strategy: Promoting High Quality Care for All Adults at the End of Life.* London: DH.

Detering, K.M., Hancock, A.D., Reade, M.C. and Silvester, W. (2010) 'The impact of advance care planning on end of life care in elderly patients: randomised controlled trial.' *British Medical Journal, 340*: 1345.

Goodrich, J., Harrison, T. and Cornwell, J. (2015) *Resilence. A Framework Supporting Hospice Staff to Flourish in Stressful Times.* London: Hospice UK.

Independent Review of the Liverpool Care Pathway (2013) *More Care, Less Pathway: A Review of The Liverpool Care Pathway.* Available at https://assets.publishing.service.gov. uk/government/uploads/system/uploads/attachment_data/file/212450/Liverpool_Care_ Pathway.pdf, accessed 4 June 2018.

Krishnan, M.S., Racsa, M. and Michael Yu, H-H (eds) (2017) *Handbook of Supportive and Palliative Radiation Oncology.* London: Elsevier.

Manitta, V.J., Philip, J. and Cole-Sinclair, M.F. (2010) 'Palliative care and the hemato-oncological patient: can we live together? A review of the literature.' *Journal of Palliative Medicine, 13* (8): 1021–5.

Marie Curie (2016) *The Hidden Challenges of Palliative Cancer Care.* London: Marie Curie.

Momen, C. and Barclay, S.I. (2011) 'Addressing "the elephant on the table": barriers to end of life care conversations in heart failure – a literature review and narrative synthesis.' *Current Opinion in Supportive and Palliative Care, 5* (4): 312–16.

Multinational Association of Supportive Care in Cancer (MASCC) (2013) *Definition of Supportive Care.* Toronto, Ontario: MASSC.

National Council for Hospice and Specialist Palliative Care Services (2002) *Definitions of Supportive and Palliative Care.* NCHSPCS.

National Institute for Health and Care Excellence (NICE) (2004) *Improving Supportive and Palliative Care for Adults with Cancer.* CSG4. London: NICE.

National Palliative and End of Life Care Partnership (2015) *Ambitions for Palliative and End of Life Care: A National Framework for Local Action 2015–2020.* Available at http://endoflifecareambitions.org.uk/wp-content/uploads/2015/09/Ambitions-for-Palliative-and-End-of-Life-Care.pdf, accessed 4 June 2018.

NHS England (2016) *Enhanced Supportive Care.* Available at www.england.nhs.uk/wp-content/uploads/2016/03/ca1-enhncd-supprtv-care-guid.pdf, accessed 4 June 2018.

Royal College of Physicians (2016) *End of life care audit-dying in hospital: National report for England 2016.* London: RCP.

Skilbeck, J.K. and Payne, S. (2005) 'End of life care: a discursive analysis of specialist palliative care nursing.' *Journal of Advanced Nursing,* 51 (4): 325–34.

Temel, J,S., Greer, J,A., Muzikansky, A., Gallagher, E.R., et al. 2010) 'Early palliative care for patients with metastatic non-small-cell lung cancer.' *New England Journal Medicine, 363*: 733–42.

World Health Organization (1990) *Cancer Pain Relief and Palliative Care: Report of a WHO Committee [Meeting Held in Geneva from 3 to 10 July 1989].* Geneva: WHO.

FURTHER READING

Bakitas, M.A., Tosteson, T.D., Li, Z., Lyons, K.D. et al. (2015) 'Early versus delayed initiation of concurrent palliative oncology care: patient outcomes in the ENABLE III randomized controlled trial.' *Journal of Clinical Oncology,* 33 (13): 1438–45.

Greer, J.A. (2012) 'Effect of early palliative care on chemotherapy use and end-of-life care in patients with metastatic non-small-cell lung cancer.' *Journal of Clinical Oncology,* 30 (4): 394–447.

12

END OF LIFE CARE IN THE COMMUNITY

ALISON NEWEY

LEARNING OUTCOMES

- Gain an understanding of the features of palliative care in the community, including recognition that a patient is reaching the end of their life
- Develop insight into the experience of carers and the support services available
- Consider the impact of effective documentation/communication
- Gain an understanding of the context of hospice and residential home care

---

INTRODUCTION

This book has focused on the provision of palliative care to patients with malignant or non-malignant medical conditions. The overarching features of this care have been discussed to give insights into areas such as pathophysiology, disease management and symptom control in relation to the patient's diagnosis. Contemporary healthcare practice also places a great deal of emphasis upon recovery from cancer and living beyond diagnosis and treatment (Independent Cancer Taskforce, 2015) while long-term conditions are better managed as medical interventions advance and improve (NHS England, 2014).

For some patients, however, there are no curative or palliative treatment options available to them as they approach an advanced stage of malignant or non-malignant disease. The aim of this chapter is to present an overview of the care provided to patients and their family members in the community setting at the end of life. The chapter describes the care of patients at the end of life with a particular focus on physical, psychological, social and spiritual factors. The services available to support patients and carers are described, providing examples of different levels of intervention. In a Cochrane systematic review, Gomes et al. (2013) propose that over 50 per cent of people would choose to die at home if the option was available to them. However, it is worth noting that the documented place of care at the end of life could incorporate hospices, residential care or nursing homes under the title of 'home'. An earlier publication by The National End of Life Care Intelligence Network (2010) illustrates the complexities of defining where patients are cared for at the end of their life with over 80 different residential or hospital settings described. In this chapter, the preferred place of care is discussed in terms of patients whose condition begins to deteriorate expressing a wish to be cared for at home, in the hospice or in residential care. An important consideration is whether the care agencies and support networks are available to provide the type of care required to meet the patient's needs (The National Council for Palliative Care, 2008).

In 2014, the Leadership Alliance for the Care of Dying People (LACDP) published guidelines with five key priorities of care (see Box 12.1). These priorities provide a structured approach, promoting good communication that includes the patient and the people caring for them. In a situation that is likely to be unfamiliar to most people, this framework can support the patient to be cared for at home and ensure that their needs, and carers' needs, are met.

BOX 12.1   FIVE PRIORITIES OF CARE (LACDP, 2014)

Priority 1: This possibility [that a person may die within the next few days or hours] is recognised and communicated clearly, decisions made and actions taken in accordance with the person's needs and wishes, and these are regularly reviewed and decisions revised accordingly.

Priority 2: Sensitive communication takes place between staff and the dying person, and those identified as important to them.

Priority 3: The dying person, and those identified as important to them, are involved in decisions about treatment and care to the extent that the dying person wants.

Priority 4: The needs of families and others identified as important to the dying person are actively explored, respected and met as far as possible.

Priority 5: An individual plan of care, which includes food and drink, symptom control and psychological, social and spiritual support, is agreed, coordinated and delivered with compassion.

REFLECTIVE EXERCISE 12.1

Spend some time looking at the priorities of care guidance in Box 12.1 (LACDP, 2014) and consider how these can help healthcare practitioners to provide good care at the end of a patient's life. How might these features empower the patient and carers to make decisions about end of life care in the community setting?

DEFINING THE END OF LIFE

The General Medical Council (2010) define 'end of life' as the last year of life, not limited to the final days before death. This perspective is reinforced by the National Gold Standards Framework (GSF) Centre (2017) with their *Going for Gold* initiative for primary care providers and the *Prognostic Indicator Guidance* (National GSF Centre, 2011). GPs are encouraged to identify all patients who have reached the palliative care phase of their illness. There is also a need to maintain a patient register to discuss care management on a regular basis, usually at multidisciplinary meetings. The Prognostic Indicator Guidance (National GSF Centre, 2011) distinguishes between different stages of the last year of life with a red, amber or green classification (Figure 12.1). It can be seen that the green phase depicts an advancing stage of disease progression, with an anticipated prognosis of approximately 12 months. As the timeline moves towards amber, there is an expectation that a patient's prognosis is likely to be thought of in terms of weeks, while the red stage reflects that the patient has a prognosis of days or less than this. Each of these stages gives an indication of the level of care that a person might require and this can structure palliative care meetings and health practitioner discussions in the primary care setting. For effective end of life care planning, the GP register should be dynamic in order to reflect when a patient's condition is changing and an appropriate level of care needs to be introduced. The Prognostic Indicator Guidance (National GSF Centre, 2011) also highlights that the care of patients with non-malignant life-limiting illness can be less predictable than the management of end-stage malignant illness which has a more linear progression. For the purposes of this chapter, the term 'end of life' will be used to discuss the delivery of patient care in the dying phase.

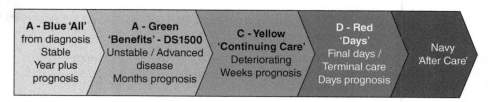

Figure 12.1

CASE STUDY 12.1 MR C

Mr C was diagnosed with advanced-stage lung cancer. While undergoing palliative chemo-therapy treatment his condition was discussed at his GP surgery using the Gold Standards Framework (National Gold Standards Framework [GSF], 2011) with the relevant healthcare pro-fessionals present – that is, GPs, district nurses, social worker and the community palliative care team. His prognosis at that stage was considered in terms of months, which was repre-sented by the 'green' phase of illness. The plan of care was therefore agreed that community nurses would monitor him on a monthly basis.

After a period of six months, Mr C received the news that his disease had progressed, despite treatment, and there were no further options available for palliative chemotherapy or radiotherapy. Mr C was becoming increasingly symptomatic with shortness of breath, fatigue and pain both at the site of the lung cancer and metastatic disease in his ribs. Previous contacts from healthcare teams had been to monitor his condition and his ability to cope with the effects of his disease. The GSF meeting discussed his advanced stage of the disease, now more relevant to the 'yellow' phase of the palliative care register. Mr C was referred to the community palliative care team for supportive care and symptom management to complement the community nursing team's input. With a joint approach from the multidisciplinary team this gentleman's care was delivered at an appropriate level for his needs and all healthcare teams were prepared for increasing their input at the end of life stage.

In recognition of the need for effective end of life care, the National Institute for Health and Care Excellence (NICE) (2017) published quality standards to guide health practitioners who care for dying patients (see Box 12.2). The standards reflect the complexity of recognising that a patient is approaching death and rein-force the message that any reversible elements of a life-limiting condition are assessed and managed appropriately for each individual.

BOX 12.2 QUALITY STANDARDS (NICE, 2017)

Standard 1: Adults who have signs and symptoms that suggest they may be in the last days of life are monitored for further changes to help determine if they are nearing death, stabilising or recovering.

Standard 2: Adults in the last days of life, and the people important to them, are given opportu-nities to discuss, develop and review an individualised care plan.

Standard 3: Adults in the last days of life who are likely to need symptom control are prescribed anticipatory medicines with individualised indications for use, dosage and route of administration.

Standard 4: Adults in the last days of life have their hydration status assessed daily, and have a discussion about the risks and benefits of hydration options.

Reproduced with permission under the terms of the NICE UK Open Content Licence

CARER SUPPORT

Within community care service provision, the multidisciplinary team comprises healthcare professionals and other allied services – for example, medical staff, nurses, occupational therapists, physiotherapists, social workers, spiritual or religious representatives and external care agencies who are commissioned by clinical commissioning groups (CCGs) to provide additional support for patients in the community. The workforce of these care agencies consists of healthcare assistants who can provide assistance with patients' personal hygiene needs, moving and handling or meals at the later stages of illness. As patients approach the end of life, these care agencies provide valuable support to families and can enable the patient to remain at home. As an emerging model of care, integration is promoted as an effective method of health and social services working synergistically in the community (Hawkins, 2011; NHS England, 2014). Integrated care as a concept is loosely defined however (Hawkes, 2013) and its true approach remains subject to debate. For the patient who is reaching the end of life, the combination of health and social care services enables care to be delivered in the home or residential setting. Figure 12.2 gives detail of the process that might be followed in order to arrange for a patient to be transferred home, to fulfil their wish to die at home.

Patients who wish to be cared for in the community are likely to be dependent on the support that their family or friends can provide as informal carers. With the use of careful communication skills, it can be determined at an opportune moment that a patient would like to document their preferred wishes at the end of life (National PPC Review Team, 2007). There are many formats available for care plans and each healthcare trust may have their own version. The decision making around a patient's preferred place of care or death may have been established in the earlier stages of disease. However, the experience of being cared for in an environment external to a hospital may also lead the patient to make changes to their decision as their disease progresses (The National Council for Palliative Care, 2008). For example, patients who experience the symptom of breathlessness might feel less frightened when they are cared for in a hospital setting (Gysels et al., 2007). Although they have previously expressed a preference to be cared for at home, their anxiety around breathlessness and fear of feeling that they are suffocating might trigger a hospital admission if this symptom is not managed effectively. Booth (2009) comments on inappropriate admissions to hospital when a breathless patient is at the end of life and outlines the circumstances whereby family or carers might call for an ambulance if they are unsure of what else they can do in this situation.

In a qualitative study of informal carers' experiences of looking after someone who is dying at home, Hudson (2004) offers a valuable insight into the fears and demands of being in this role. In particular, carers expressed worries about the weight of expectation placed upon them and frustration at being confined to the home with little opportunity to go out at all. Interestingly, the interviews also

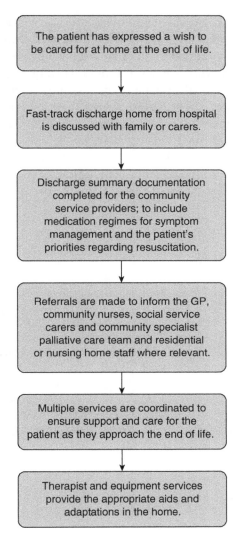

Figure 12.2   Features of care planning for patients discharged from acute care at the end of life

revealed that over a third of those who took part in the study had felt uncomfortable due to not having the skills to manage symptoms, which might suggest more of a gap in healthcare practitioners' support than the carers' abilities.

An assessment of the patient's social circumstances and the demands placed upon their carers can highlight a need for additional care agency input (Stajduhar, 2013). Social care is an intrinsic factor in assessing a patient and their carers for community-based care. As discussed in an earlier section, external agency care support can be drawn upon, if needed, to give family or carers the opportunity to rest or to spend some time away from their responsibilities in the home. Local health organisations (CCGs) can provide continuing healthcare (NHS Choices, 2015) to support full-time care based on a primary health need. Continuing healthcare recognises that the patient is entitled to care that is funded by the State and the support usually comprises carers who visit several times daily, or as needed for each individual, to assist with personal hygiene needs and any other care required. Social services care agency input can be set up promptly for any patient who is reaching the end of life and requires additional support, although the increased number of staff coming into the home on a frequent basis can be a shortcoming of this option for some families. To illustrate this point further, Case study 12.2 illustrates the social care input and the notion of continuing healthcare that enables patients to be discharged from hospital to home at the end of life.

CASE STUDY 12.2   JANE

Jane was reaching the end of her life and had been referred to the community specialist palliative care team for symptom management and to provide psychological support for her and her family. Community nurses were already caring for this lady and providing daily visits to assess her condition and general care needs. When additional visits were introduced by the palliative care team it was evident that this was intrusive and difficult for Jane's husband Bill as he came to terms with his wife's deteriorating health. For this family, it was important to keep services to a minimum. The community nurses therefore maintained their daily contacts with Jane while liaising with the GP and community specialist palliative care team for guidance or support with any complex areas of symptom management. The most important feature for Jane was that she was comfortable at home and cared for in a way that suited her and her family.

SYMPTOM MANAGEMENT/CARER FATIGUE/CARER BREAKDOWN

Care of patients at the end of life requires dynamic assessment of individual symptoms and an anticipatory approach towards managing these; thus the community setting can offer the patient comfort in being cared for in a familiar environment with the people around them who are important to them (Gomes and Higginson, 2006). Various community services, such as GP, community nurses, palliative care nurses, community specialist physiotherapist and occupational therapist, care agencies, night-carer services and complementary therapists are called upon to provide clinical nursing care, essential care, therapy support, symptom management, befriending and psychological support as determined by the patient's individual needs. Home visits are arranged by each service according to the needs of the patient. In between these visits, however, great responsibility is placed upon informal carers to maintain patient care and observation. Informal carers are required to carry on the usual daily activities of the home and to respond to the patient's needs, all of which places a great responsibility upon family or friends (Stajduhar, 2013). For example, the informal carer is likely to be required to oversee the administration of prescribed medication and to be aware of when to contact health or social care services for advice.

Hudson (2004) highlights the positive features and difficulties of the informal carer role when caring for a dying relative or friend. Initially, these informal carers may not have any insight into the demands of the role that they willingly or unwittingly have adopted, and the potential for carer breakdown should be considered when assessing the patient in the community setting. An additional factor may be that the carer's relationship with the patient was already under strain prior to illness developing, leading to difficulties when undertaking an informal carer role.

The needs of the family are an intrinsic element of the holistic patient assessment and the introduction of additional supportive care from community services should complement the ability of the carers to cope with a demanding situation that may have an impact upon their lives long after the patient has died. In a Cochrane review of the effectiveness of home care at the end of life, Gomes et al. (2013) reported that family or friend care providers who are supported by community palliative care services do not experience any increased effect on their grief when a relative dies at home. Bakitas and Dionne-Odom (2017) contest this consideration, however, with a reminder that the death of a relative in the home may leave family or close friends struggling with difficult recollections of the event. In situations where carers feel that they are no longer able to continue as the main carer for the patient, additional services can be introduced to offset the effects of sleep deprivation and perceived social isolation (Stajduhar, 2013). Sitting or befriending services can augment the support that an informal carer can provide, allowing them to spend time away from the caring situation and an opportunity to sleep while the patient is accompanied. Support services are provided by charitable organisations such as Marie Curie, Age UK or local volunteer agencies. It is the role of community nurses or the palliative care team to assess the need for support and to coordinate these services to suit the patient and their family.

COMMUNICATION

This chapter thus far has demonstrated that there are multiple services responsible for delivering care at the end of life in the community setting – GPs, community nurses, palliative care nurses, allied health professionals, social workers, agency care workers, complementary therapists, voluntary services, hospices and members of religious or spiritual doctrines may all play a part in a patient's care. The underpinning feature of effective patient care is good communication (LACDP, 2014). The LACDP (2014) document clearly states that within this extended multidisciplinary team there needs to be a robust method of sharing information and ensuring that everyone is kept fully informed of the patient's individual plan of care. Media reports of poor standards of care for patients at the end of life led to a UK Government Inquiry (Department of Health and Social Care, 2013), which reported a lack of shared information between patients, their families and people close to them, care providers and healthcare professionals.

Healthcare practitioners might feel that they do not have the skills or time to respond to a patient or others' cues/questions about the plan of care. An opportunity to explore fears, thoughts and feelings may therefore be missed. Box 12.1 above demonstrates a theme of communication running throughout its key points, with an emphasis upon ensuring that all people involved in a patient's care are kept fully informed. The families and carers of patients may not have been exposed to a situation before where a person is reaching the end of life stages and, often, they do not know what to expect. Acknowledgement by a medical professional that a person is dying is an important aspect of care; it allows the patient, and those close to them, an opportunity to ask questions and to consider any unresolved issues in their lives.

Often, a community palliative care nurse can facilitate conversations between family members, carers and the patient by using specialist communication skills and careful listening techniques. In the community, patient care plans are documented in the residential setting. Following the decommissioning of the Liverpool Care Pathway (LACDP, 2014), individual local organisations have designed different ways of coordinating and documenting patient care during the last days of life. Alongside the notes kept in the patient's home there may be a record of their preferred wishes in an advance care plan (ACP). Establishing these preferred wishes is a sensitive issue that requires careful communication skills (The National Council for Palliative Care, 2008; LACDP, 2014); patients may intimate that they would like to discuss their thoughts and a careful listener will pick up on this during conversation.

The National Council for Palliative Care (2008) and LACDP (2014) emphasise the importance of giving patients the opportunity to have these discussions while they have the legally determined mental capacity (NHS Choices, 2018) to make their own decisions. Bakitas and Dionne-Odom (2017) discuss the importance of knowing what a patient's wishes are, especially if a situation arises where hospital admission is being considered. Admissions to the acute care setting can be minimised when families and carers are aware of a patient's preferred place of care or death; this is described by The National Council for Palliative Care (2008). The value of advance care plans is optimised by ensuring that this information is shared between other care providers; the patient needs to be assessed as having mental capacity (NHS Choices, 2018) to consent to their information being shared with other teams and people involved in their care. Thus, a copy of their wishes can be provided for their GP, community nurses, out-of-hours GP services and the palliative care team.

SPECIALIST CARE AT THE END OF LIFE

Community nursing care is provided collectively by community nurses, palliative care nurses and other related specialist healthcare professionals, such as physiotherapists, occupational therapists, dieticians, speech and language teams, and social work and healthcare agency providers. For patients with a cancer diagnosis, there is an anticipated decline in functional capacity as the disease progresses; however, this decline is less predictable in long-term conditions – for example, chronic obstructive pulmonary disease, heart failure (see Chapter 2), or motor neurone disease (National GSF Centre, 2011; see Chapter 4). The focus of care for all life-limiting disease is to manage symptoms and maintain comfort, particularly at the end of life (Twycross and Wilcock, 2001). Twycross and Wilcock (2001) emphasise that a realistic approach should be taken towards symptom management, however, and the patient and carers should be aware that nurses will need to initiate treatments and review them frequently until symptoms are optimally managed. In a qualitative study of carers' experiences of looking after family or friends at the end of life, Hudson (2004) described a theme that emerged with some interviewees saying that they felt ill-equipped to deal with symptoms and in some cases felt they were not adequately supported by the healthcare teams involved. Unlike hospital-based healthcare, the nurse or allied community professional will not be present at all times. Therefore, there needs to be a clear plan of care in place, to ensure that the carers know what or who to contact if problems arise. This can be achieved by maintaining a patient-held record at the home, detailing a care plan, risk assessment for pressure area care and a record of all teams that are involved in the patient's care.

In a review of palliative nursing care, Finucane et al. (2014) described pain, breathlessness, anxiety, respiratory secretions and nausea as the symptoms most often treated at the end of life. Twycross and Wilcock (2001) advocate a pragmatic approach towards addressing symptoms at the end of life and recommend that different approaches, both pharmacological and non-pharmacological, should be adopted to maintain the patient's comfort. Community nursing teams are responsible for regularly visiting the patient, to assess symptoms and to review the effectiveness of the care being provided. Pharmacological management of pain, nausea, vomiting, restlessness or breathlessness is usually addressed by the patient's GP who will prescribe medication for symptom management; in some organisations it may also be a non-medical prescriber who can issue a prescription for medications to be used at the end of life. Anticipatory prescribing can ensure that medications are more readily available when the patient needs them, especially during out-of-hours periods (Griggs, 2010; Finucane et al., 2014). To minimise the potential for drugs to be abused, the storage of controlled drugs in the patient's home and recording of the administration of these will be managed according to local pharmacy policy.

In the community setting, nurses attending a patient will use their clinical judgement to decide which medications to introduce into the plan of care and also decide on the most suitable route of administration for that person. In a qualitative study of community nurses' experiences of making these clinical judgements, Wilson et al. (2015) provide valuable insights into the complexities that nurses face when caring for a patient at the end of life and the ethical dilemmas that arise when administering medications for the purpose of symptom control. Community nurses provide care both for the patient and also those close to them at a sensitive time; the use of powerful medications at the end of life precedes the death of the patient and can be construed as shortening their life in some instances. Registered community nurses work to a prescribed dosage range of medicines for the management of symptoms and are required to make a clinical judgement to address symptoms, such as pain, vomiting or agitation. With support from the specialist palliative care team or GP, the community nurse can assess the need to alter doses administered or to commence medications via a continuous subcutaneous syringe driver to suit the patient's condition. Anecdotally, the introduction of a syringe driver can be unsettling to some relatives or friends and will need sensitive discussion to demonstrate where its use is in the best interests of the patient.

This chapter has discussed that the management and control of a patient's physical symptoms frequently requires the use of controlled drugs. The use of potent groups of medicines such as opioids and benzodiazepines can address pain and agitation; however, there may be an unwanted outcome of administering such powerful medications. The concept of 'double effect' (Twycross and Wilcock, 2001; Allmark et al., 2010) is contentious for community nurses. Twycross and Wilcock (2001) caution that medication should be used judiciously to maintain comfort while avoiding euthanasia. Allmark et al. (2010) contend that 'double effect' does not reflect a 'bad' outcome for the dying patient and thus is not a doctrine in the context of end of life care. The study by Wilson et al. (2015) outlines the pressure and responsibilities that community nurses are subject to when making decisions around end of life symptom control and the authors recommend a joint approach between health practitioners to share the burden of decision making. Anticipatory prescribing of medications for symptom management has a place in the care of patients at the end of life (Finucane et al., 2014). However, there should also be consideration of non-pharmacological approaches that can complement the use of medications. The impact of positioning, careful touch and reassurance is recognised by Twycross and Wilcock (2001) who suggest non-pharmacological management approaches that can be incorporated into the treatment of various symptoms. Listening to patients' stories is highlighted by Kearsley (2010) as a feature of 'compassionate solidarity' between the health practitioner and the patient. Kearsley (2010) discusses the existential suffering of patients, even when they are symptom-free, and urges health practitioners to be mindful of the therapeutic effects of simply being with the patient and their carers when hope feels absent.

Therapist interventions for the patient delivered by allied health practitioners are an adjunct to carer and nursing support at the end of life. Although the focus of care is not aimed at rehabilitation, the therapy team can assess for any interventions, aids or adaptations that can offer comfort and the ability to set realistic objectives – for example, around mobility, energy conservation and coping strategies (National End of Life Care Programme, 2011). The National End of Life Care Programme (2011) also mirrors the Six Steps initiative discussed in more detail below.

RESIDENTIAL CARE

Contemporary healthcare aims to record where patients are cared for at the end of life and to measure this against where they had expressed that they wanted to be. Interpretation of data around patients who die in their preferred place should incorporate people who are in residential care, however, and thus class this as their home. The term 'residential care' covers nursing homes, care homes and could also encompass the hospice setting (De Roo et al., 2014). Within care and nursing homes the majority of the workforce is likely to consist of unregistered health workers who have cared for residents in the home for long periods of time. The staff are therefore likely to be familiar with the patient's needs and also their family or friends. When the patient reaches the end of life phase, their care can be managed in the residential setting with support from the GP and community services if needed. Community nurses can review patients who are in care homes while hospice care is provided by a multidisciplinary team of medical staff, qualified nurses and therapists along with healthcare assistants. DeRoo et al. (2014) argue that although performance indicators can demonstrate when patients have died in their preferred place of care, these do not reflect the quality of the end of life care received. In some organisations, additional training and support is available for care home staff to deliver effective end of life care, particularly where there is a lack of experience in recognising the end of life phase (Unroe et al., 2015).

The Six Steps Programme of Care (Cheshire & Merseyside Clinical Network and Greater Manchester, Lancashire & South Cumbria Clinical Network, 2017) is a strategy for supporting care home staff in the delivery of end of life care, aiming to reduce unnecessary transfers to hospital and encouraging appropriate management of the end of life phase. The programme follows the *GSF Prognostic Indicator Guidance* (National Gold Standard Framework Centre, 2011) and encourages care homes to maintain a register of their patients who require palliative care. As the end of life approaches, patients' symptoms can be managed with effective care planning. Health workers can pre-empt the opportunity to discuss preferences for care at the end of life (National Council for Palliative Care, 2008). For patients who do not have the mental capacity to make their own decisions about their care, a 'best interests' meeting can be held on their behalf (National Council for Palliative Care, 2008). These meetings are equivalent across community settings, however, and can take place at the patient's own home, GP surgery, hospice or within the residential care home. Best interest meetings represent a formal procedure whereby the multidisciplinary team members discuss all the details of a patient's situation and aim to make a decision for treatment on behalf that person (NHS Choices, 2018). The decision takes into account any preferences that a patient legally documented while they had the mental capacity to do so with regard to their care.

CASE STUDY 12.3   A CARER'S EXPERIENCE

Looking back, the experience of caring for our dad at home was a difficult time for my brother and me but probably not for him. With little knowledge of the services available to us, we dealt with each day as it arrived and tried to alleviate Dad's symptoms of pain and fatigue with minimal input from healthcare services which was his preference. However, on the occasions when we asked for guidance, we found the GP, district nurses and Macmillan team to be sadly lacking in providing us with support. None of these services was forthcoming in treating pain effectively and the main source of palliative care was from the hospital or hospice teams. Inevitably, Dad's condition deteriorated during a second line of chemotherapy treatment and he was no longer able to tolerate its side effects.

    We had the support of the local hospice outpatient clinic who monitored and supported Dad, although it was clear that he did not want to discuss his prognosis or the future; we thought he was being unrealistic in talking about 'getting better' but with hindsight, this was his way of coping with the situation. As his symptoms of abdominal distension (due to his gall bladder cancer), pain and fatigue progressed, Dad had frequent admissions to hospital. He did not want to broach the subject of death or dying, and there was no advance care plan in place, thus we felt compelled to seek secondary care review each time his condition worsened significantly. Ultimately, Dad died peacefully and comfortably in hospital with his family around him, although he had not wanted to go in on that occasion. The most credible example of care was from the out-of-hours locum GP who saw Dad on the day before he died. His quiet and assured presence gave comfort to my brother and me and reassured Dad that he should be reviewed in hospital for more comprehensive pain control. Although we had cared for Dad at home for the majority of the time that he was unwell, it did feel like he had had a good death and was settled at the time of dying, which we are grateful for.

BEREAVEMENT AND AFTERCARE

The care of a relative or friend at the end of life can have lasting repercussions for the informal carer and their ability to grieve for the loss of their relationship with that person (Stajduhar, 2013). In a study of carers' experiences of caring for a person at home, Stajduhar (2013) illuminates the feelings that can emanate from this and talks about the 'disruption' of their usual life that has occurred. Besides the psychological impact of having been in a demanding, caring role, Stajduhar (2013) also suggests that there may also be financial implications or loss of employment that can result from the disruption that is experienced during the caregiving episode. Thomas et al. (2014) conclude that the support of community palliative care services during the end of life phase can have a positive effect on carers' grief. They advocate, however, that carers should also be assessed for factors that may be associated with a difficult bereavement process that could affect them long after the patient has died – for example, feelings of hopelessness, anger or resentment when looking after the patient.

The National Gold Standards Framework (National Gold Standards Framework Centre, 2011) includes bereavement support for the patient's family or friends as a progression of the care provided by community healthcare teams. In this respect, community palliative care teams are well placed to provide support to the people who were close to a patient by contacting them at an appropriate time or making a bereavement visit, to listen to their feelings and introduce specialist bereavement therapy. Milberg et al. (2008) outline the positive effect of health practitioners contacting the patient's family or friends in their bereavement. Furthermore, a meeting between healthcare teams can be a valuable opportunity to discuss the care of a patient, particularly if there have been complex issues during the end of life management; community palliative care teams can facilitate these meetings and review the features of care that were effective or difficult to manage.

CONCLUSION

End of life care in the community setting is provided by a team of informal carers and health practitioners; the emphasis is to maintain patient comfort and dignity in the most appropriate environment for that person's care. In primary care, the National GSF Centre's (2011) *Prognostic Indicator Guidance* gives direction for assessing the stage of illness that a patient has reached and the level of palliative care that should be considered, while indicating that the continuum of care extends to bereavement support and signposting to specialist support networks. Individual patient scenarios can present a need for complex care planning that incorporates the management of physical, psychological, social and spiritual factors and ensures effective communication between all parties.

REFERENCES

Allmark, P., Cobb, M., Liddle, J. and Tod, A. (2010) 'Is the doctrine of double effect irrelevant in end-of-life decision making?' *Nursing Philosophy*, 11: 170–7.

Bakitas, M. and Dionne-Odom, J.N. (2017) 'When it comes to death, there's no place like home... or is there?' *Palliative Medicine*, 31 (5): 391–3.

Booth, S. (2009) 'End of life care for the breathless patient.' *General Practice Update*, 2 (1): 40–4.

Cheshire & Merseyside Clinical Network and Greater Manchester, Lancashire & South Cumbria Clinical Network (2017) *Six Steps to Success in End of Life Care*. Available at www.sixsteps.net, accessed 4 June 2018.

Department of Health and Social Care (2013) *Mid Staffordshire NHS FT public inquiry: government response*. Available at https://www.gov.uk/government/publications/mid-staffordshire-nhs-ft-public-inquiry-government-response, accessed 26 June 2018.

De Roo, M.L., Miccinesi, G., Onwuteaka-Philipsen, B.D., Van Den Noortgate, N., et al. (2014) 'Actual and preferred place of death of home-dwelling patients in four European countries: making sense of quality indicators.' *Public Library of Science ONE*, 9 (4): e93762.

Finucane, A., McArthur, D., Stevenson, B., Gardner, H. and Murray, S. (2014) 'Anticipatory prescribing at the end of life in Lothian care homes.' *British Journal of Community Nursing, 19* (11): 544–7.

General Medical Council (2010) *Treatment and Care towards the End of Life: Good Practice in Decision-Making.* Available from: www.gmc-uk.org/static/documents/content/Treatment_and_care_towards_the_end_of_life_-_English_1015.pdf, accessed 11 April 2017.

Gomes, B. and Higginson, I. (2006) 'Factors influencing death at home in terminally ill patients with cancer: systematic review.' *BMJ, 332* (7450): 515–21.

Gomes, B., Calanzani, N., Curiale, V., McCrone, P. and Higginson, I.J. (2013) 'Effectiveness and cost-effectiveness of home palliative care services for adults with advanced illness and their caregivers.' *The Cochrane Database of Systematic Reviews 6* June (6): CD007760.

Griggs, C. (2010) 'Community nurses' perceptions of a good death: a qualitative exploratory study.' *International Journal of Palliative Nursing, 16* (3): 140–8.

Gysels, M., Bausewein, C. and Higginson, I. (2007) 'Experiences of breathlessness: a systematic review of the qualitative literature.' *Palliative and Supportive Care, 5* (3): 281–302.

Hawkes, N. (2013) 'Take me to your leader.' *BMJ, 346:* f2092.

Hawkins, L. (2011) *Can Competition and Integration Co-exist in a Reformed NHS?* London: The King's Fund. Available at www.kingsfund.org.uk/publications/can-competition-and-integration-co-exist-reformed-nhs, accessed 29 April 2017.

Hudson, P. (2004) 'Positive aspects and challenges associated with caring for a dying relative at home.' *International Journal of Palliative Care Nursing, 10* (2), 58–65.

Independent Cancer Taskforce (2015) *Achieving World Class Cancer Outcomes: A Strategy for England, 2015–2020.* Available at www.cancerresearchuk.org/sites/default/files/achieving_world-class_cancer_outcomes_-_a_strategy_for_england_2015-2020.pdf, accessed 4 April 2017.

Kearsley, J. (2010) 'Therapeutic use of self and the relief of suffering.' *Cancer Forum, 34* (2): 71–4.

Leadership Alliance for the Care of the Dying Person (LACDP) (2014) *One Chance to Get It Right.* Available at www.gov.uk/government/uploads/system/uploads/attachment_data/file/323188/One_chance_to_get_it_right.pdf, accessed 6 April 2017.

Milberg, A., Olsson, E., Jacobson, M., Olsson, M. and Friedrichsen, M. (2008) 'Family members' perceived needs for bereavement follow-up.' *Journal of Pain and Symptom Management, 35* (1): 58–69.

National Council for Palliative Care (2008) *Advance Care Planning: A Guide for Health and Social Care Staff.* Available at www.ncpc.org.uk/sites/default/files/AdvanceCarePlanning.pdf, accessed 19 April 2017.

National End of Life Care Intelligence Network (2010) *Variations in Place of Death.* Available at www.endoflifecare-intelligence.org.uk/search/variations+in+place+of+death, accessed 25 April 2017.

National End of Life Care Programme (2011) *The Route to Success in End of Life Care – Achieving Quality for Occupational Therapy.* Available at www.leedspalliativecare.co.uk/wp-content/uploads/2014/05/rts_ot___final_web_version___20110627-1.pdf, accessed 1 May 2017.

National Gold Standards Framework (GSF) Centre (2011) *The GSF Prognostic Indicator Guidance.* Available at www.goldstandardsframework.org.uk/cd-content/uploads/files/General%20Files/Prognostic%20Indicator%20Guidance%20October%202011.pdf, accessed 11 April 2017.

National Gold Standards Framework (GSF) Centre (2017) *Going for Gold.* Available at http://www.goldstandardsframework.org.uk/primary-care-training-programme, accessed 11 April 2017.

National Institute for Health and Care Excellence (NICE) (2017) *Care of Dying Adults in the Last Days of Life*. QS144. London: NICE. Available at www.nice.org.uk/guidance/QS144/chapter/quality-statements, accessed 17 April 2017.

National PPC Review Team (2007) *Preferred Priorities for Care*. Available at www.dyingmatters.org/sites/default/files/preferred_priorities_for_care.pdf, accessed 4 June 2018.

NHS Choices (2015) *NHS Continuing Healthcare*. Available at www.nhs.uk/Conditions/social-care-and-support-guide/Pages/nhs-continuing-care.aspx, accessed 20 April 2017.

NHS Choices (2018) *What is the Mental Capacity Act?* Available at www.nhs.uk/conditions/social-care-and-support/mental-capacity/#is-the-decision-in-their-best-interests, accessed 26 June 2018.

NHS England (2014) *Five Year Forward View*. Available at www.england.nhs.uk/wp-content/uploads/2014/10/5yfv-web.pdf, accessed 29 April 2017.

Stajduhar, K. (2013) 'Burdens of family caregiving at the end of life.' *Clinical & Investigative Medicine*, 36 (3): E121–6.

Thomas, K., Hudson, P., Trauer, T., Remedios, C. and Clarke, D. (2014) 'Risk factors for developing prolonged grief during bereavement in family carers of cancer patients in palliative care: a longitudinal study.' *Journal of Pain and Symptom Management*, 47 (3): 531–41.

Twycross, R. and Wilcock, A. (2001) *Symptom Management in Advanced Cancer*. 3rd ed. Nottingham: Palliativedrugs.com.

Unroe, K., Cagle, J., Lane, K., Callahan, C. and Miller, S. (2015) 'Nursing home staff palliative care knowledge and practices: results of a large survey of frontline workers.' *Journal of Pain and Symptom Management*, 50 (5): 622–9.

Wilson, A., Morbey, H., Brown, J., Payne, S., Seale, C. and Seymour, J. (2015) 'Administering anticipatory medications in end of life care: a qualitative study of nursing practice in the community and in nursing homes.' *Palliative Medicine*, 29 (1): 60–70.

FURTHER READING

National End of Life Care Programme (2012) *The Route to Success in End of Life Care – Achieving Quality for Lesbian, Gay, Bisexual and Transgender People*. Available at www.macmillan.org.uk/documents/aboutus/health_professionals/endoflifecare-lgbtroutetosuccess.pdf, accessed 13 February 2017.

CONCLUSION: THE CASE STUDY APPROACH

The book has taken a non-traditional stance in many ways by reaching out to embrace the care and treatment of people with non-cancer medical conditions that require palliative care. The call for palliative care to consider medical conditions other than cancer stems from the early 1990s and it has taken nearly two decades for this to start to become a reality. This book is rather unique, not only because it includes chapters on end stage medical conditions but it has a chapter written by a patient still receiving treatment. Moreover, most of the writers are clinicians and people who are close to the bedside as well as those in close contact with families and lay caregivers. The two parts of the book reflect a distinction in their approach. Part I focuses on the key requirement of palliative care practitioners to have knowledge and understanding of the patient's illness trajectory and pathophysiology. Part II focuses more on the support services available to help practitioners become informed and implement quality care. Using the term support services does not denote a lesser importance, as all services are aware of the need to work well together to ensure positive patient experiences.

The book, however, has maintained traditional approaches and understandings to palliative care by paying attention to lay caregivers, some of whom are family members. The contribution made by caregivers, as the book stipulates, is enormous and is often made at great personal cost to emotional wellbeing.

In order to achieve its aim of raising awareness about the experiences of families and patients on the palliative care journey, the book has extensively used case studies. Many of these are real-life examples and focus on real problems encountered by the chapter writers. The book has used case studies for several reasons; first they enable writers to share their experiences of caring for people with a life limiting illness. At the same time they add credibility to the text because, the reader is able to consider how many of the theoretical models cited can be implemented in practice. A less considered reason is the therapeutic effect case studies can have on the patient and family. Case studies can and do enrich the experiences of patients and caregivers. They do this by facilitating the sharing of life experiences. This, in itself, can have a cathartic effect; encouraging the patient and caregiver to make public what they have encountered during their palliative journey (Burns et al 2007).

Consider some of the key experiences in the chapters, for example Kenneth's story in Chapter 4 and Joan's experiences in Chapters 1 and 5. These case studies represent the life experiences of real people, consider the story of David and Anne in Chapter 8. Their case studies then reflect a reality seen by the authors of the chapters, presented in the book for the reader. The case studies then are a central part of the book and their inclusion helps to amplify and enrich the experiences of the patient, practitioners, family and friends. We are grateful to the patients and families who granted us permission to use their stories. I hope that educators can perhaps utilise the case studies as teaching aids in the teaching and learning about palliative care practice.

For the reader, it is hoped that the amplification of the patient voice and their family's are useful learning tools that supplement the more theoretical, evidence-based practice core of the book.

Another central message of the book is the principle of palliative care teamwork. This has been a consistent theme throughout the chapters and all of the contributors make significant reference to the importance of teamwork in achieving palliative care goals and ensuring high quality end of life care. It is important for practitioners in hospital to be aware of the role of the hospital palliative care team, the spiritual care team and the contributions made by the social worker and the primary care team. If you take away anything from the book, it should be that teamwork is core to effective palliative care.

In addition to teamwork, four other major themes are explored in the book. The first is communication, an area with which many palliative care practitioners struggle. Second, central to developing good relationships with the patient and family is effective medical intervention to manage symptoms. Third, there is the need for advance care planning (ACP). The final theme of the book is its focus on death, dying and bereavement. All chapters make the point that palliative care is not just about quality of life but the quality of death and dying also. Dying well is a professional ideal and wherever possible, practitioners strive to ensure that patients, families and professionals experience a good death. In essence this is arguably what palliative care is about, living well and dying well.

REFERENCE

Burns, M., Costello, J., Ryan-Woolley, B. and Davidson, S. (2007) 'Assessing the impact of late treatment effects in cervical cancer: an exploratory study of women's sexuality.' *European Journal of Cancer Care*, 16: 364a–372.

GLOSSARY OF TERMS

Adjuvants: Also referred to as co-analgesics, they help to complement the effect of opioids. Some examples are antidepressants and anticonvulsants.

Advance care planning (ACP): Also referred to as future care planning, ACP is a process of reflection on, and communication and documentation of a person's future healthcare wishes.

Advanced decision: Also known as a living will, or advanced decision to refuse treatment (ADRT), an ADRT is a decision you can make before end of life to refuse a specific type of treatment at some time in the future.

Allogeneic: Stem cell transplant using donated stem cells.

Anticipatory prescribing: Prescribing medications that can alleviate symptoms when patients are dying.

Arrhythmia: An abnormal heart rhythm causing the heart to beat too slowly, too fast or irregularly.

Arteriovenous fistula (AVF): A connection between an artery and a vein, carried out by surgical intervention and created for haemodialysis treatments. The AVF is normally created in the arm and two needles are inserted into the fistula which are then connected to a haemodialysis machine.

Ascites: An abnormal accumulation of fluid in the abdomen that can cause weight gain, abdominal distension and abdominal discomfort.

Atrial fibrillation: An abnormal heart rhythm caused by extra electrical impulses from the top chambers of the heart (atria) firing in a disorganised way causing an irregular heartbeat.

Attendance allowance: Payment made to people aged 65 and over regardless of income, savings or National Insurance contribution record and is a tax-free benefit. The payment is made for people with care needs. Caregivers with care needs can also claim attendance allowance for themselves which does not affect carer's allowance.

Autologous transplant: Stem cell transplant using the patient's own stem cells.

Automated peritoneal dialysis (APD): APD works in the same way as continuous ambulatory peritoneal dialysis (CAPD). The difference is that fluid exchanges are all done at night, leaving the daytime free.

Autonomy: Key ethical principle – a person's right to make their own decisions.

Background pain: Constant, persistent pain that is experienced for more than 12 hours a day.

Basal crepitations: A cracking or crunching sound heard at the base of the lungs using a stethoscope.

Bence Jones test: A urine sample test for Bence Jones protein or free light chains where the body produces antibodies that are incomplete. The presence of any Bence Jones protein in urine is abnormal. Presence of this protein is an indicator of myeloma.

Beneficence: Key ethical principle – a moral obligation to act for the benefit of others.

Best interest decision: Related largely to people who have advanced dementia. The principle is that people with dementia should be supported to make as many decisions as they can make about their money. Best interest decisions should be made by others only when a person has been assessed as lacking capacity to make some financial decisions themselves.

Bisphosphates: A class of drugs that prevent the loss of bone density, used to treat osteoporosis and similar diseases. They are the most commonly prescribed drugs used to treat osteoporosis. An example is zoledronic acid.

Breakthrough pain: A transient exacerbation of pain which occurs either spontaneously or in relation to a specific trigger in someone who has mainly stable or adequately relieved background pain.

Buprenorphine patches: An opiate analgesic prescribed as a patch used to relieve severe pain in people who are expected to need pain medication around the clock for a long time and who cannot be treated with other medications.

Cancer induced cachexia (CIC): CIC occurs in patients with advanced cancer and may account for up to 20 per cent of deaths in cancer patients. Cachexia includes distinct metabolic changes that are the result of an acute-phase response mounted by the host as a reaction to tumour cells.

Cardiac Resynchronisation Therapy: A medical device (pacemaker) used in heart failure that is implanted to resynchronise the contractions of the heart's ventricles by sending electrical impulses to the heart muscle to maximise the pumping action of the heart.

Carer's allowance: The main welfare benefit to help carers. Caregivers do not have to be related to or live with the person they care for to claim carer's allowance.

Cast nephropathy: The formation of plugs (urinary casts) in the renal tubules from free immunoglobulin light chains leading to renal failure in the context of multiple myeloma.

Categorical imperative: Moral law that is unconditional or absolute for all agents.

Cheyne stoke breathing: Referred to as Cheyne stoking, this is an abnormal pattern of breathing characterised by progressively deeper, and sometimes faster, breathing followed by a gradual decrease that results in a temporary stop in breathing called an apnoea. The pattern repeats, with each cycle usually taking 30 seconds to two minutes.

Clinical commissioning groups (CCGs): clinically-led statutory NHS bodies responsible for the planning and commissioning of healthcare services for their local area.

Complementary therapy (CAMS): Non-pharmaceutical interventions for the benefit of patient care – e.g. relaxation therapy, massage or acupuncture.

Conjugal grief: Grief resulting from the loss of a spouse, considered to be one of the most difficult psychological and social issues through which someone can pass.

Consequentialism (utilitarianism): Main ethical theory focusing on the rightness or wrongness of the consequences of a person's actions to promote the greatest good.

Continuing bonds: Often referred to as continuing bonds theory, this refers to an aspect of the bereavement process which challenges the popular model of grief requiring the bereaved to 'let go' of or detach from the deceased. In contrast, continuing bonds theory advocates maintaining a spiritual attachment to the deceased as a healthy way of coping with loss.

Continuing healthcare funding: Financial assistance for people with a primary health need provided by the NHS if the patient is in a hospice, care home or their own home. In England, the NHS can arrange care for the patient or a named person as a direct payment, known as a personal health budget.

Continuous ambulatory peritoneal dialysis (CAPD): The most portable type of dialysis, CAPD uses manual bags containing peritoneal dialysis fluid. Usually carried out daily, via peritoneal cavity, with bag changes four times a day.

CRAB: Shorthand for diagnosing myeloma where raised calcium, renal impairment, anaemia and bone lesions or fractures are present.

Cyclophosphamide: Chemotherapy drug used in combination with other drugs as part of cancer treatment.

Deontology: Main ethical theory focusing on the rightness or wrongness of actions themselves.

Dexamethasone: Steroid used in combination with other drugs as part of chemotherapy treatment.

Direct payment budget: A direct payment is paid to the patient by the local council to help to meet their support.

Do Not Actively Resuscitate orders (DNAR): A medical instruction not to carry out cardiopulmonary resuscitation (CPR) if a patient's breathing stops or if the patient's heart stops beating.

DSS 1500: A document that enables attendance allowance, personal independence payment, and employment and support allowance to be claimed as benefits for the terminally ill. The form is available from a doctor, specialist or consultant. It is not necessary to see the doctor to obtain the report.

Dysarthria: Caused by paralysis, weakness or inability to coordinate the muscles of the mouth. May be a sign of a neuromuscular disorder such as cerebral palsy, Parkinson's disease or multiple sclerosis (MS).

Echocardiogram: An ultrasound scan to review the pumping action, valves, size and structure of the heart.

End of life care: Can mean any period from the last year of life of a person with a chronic and progressive disease, to the last hours or days of life. Encompasses both supportive and palliative care.

End stage pulmonary disease (ESPD): A complex and variable illness characterised by long-term deterioration of the respiratory system, leading to a diminished ability to breathe.

Enhanced supportive care in cancer: New model of collaborative working with clinicians to promote the integration of early palliative care.

Erythropoietin (EPO): An injection used to treat anaemia by stimulating production of haemoglobin to increase red blood cell count.

Euthanasia: The act of deliberately ending a person's life to relieve suffering.

Fungating tumour: The (ulcerating) wounds that develop when cancer breaks through the skin.

Generic palliative care: Adoption of the palliative care approach by the workforce, which focuses on quality of life using a whole-person or holistic approach.

Gold Standards Framework (GSF end of life care): National training and coordinating centre for providing a gold standard of care for people nearing the end of life.

Good death: A concept in palliative care, good deaths are considered to be the best death that can be achieved in the context of the individual's clinical diagnosis and symptoms, as well as the specific social, cultural and spiritual circumstances, taking into account the patient's and carer's wishes and professional expertise.

Grief work: A term used in bereavement to emphasise that grief is a process that we engage in as active participants. Grief work is emotional in nature and requires that the bereaved work through individual emotional problems to achieve resolution of their grief.

Haemodialysis: A method of removing waste products and extra fluid that build up in the blood in renal failure. Blood is pumped out of the body to an artificial kidney machine and is returned by tubes connected to the machine.

Haemopoietic cancers: Cancers that affect the blood, bone marrow, lymph and lymphatic system.

Haldane effect: This occurs when oxygenation of blood in the lungs displaces carbon dioxide from haemoglobin, which increases the removal of carbon dioxide. Conversely, oxygenated blood has a reduced affinity for carbon dioxide.

Hickman line: A central venous catheter most often used for the administration of chemotherapy or other medications, as well as for the withdrawal of blood for analysis.

Hippocratic oath: An oath written by Hippocrates – physicians should treat patients to the best of their ability and do no harm.

Hospice UK: A national charity for hospice care, supporting over 200 hospices in the UK.

Hospital palliative care teams: Specialist palliative care professionals working in district general hospitals or cancer centres alongside an oncology team.

Hypercalcaemia: A high calcium level in the blood serum. The normal range is 2.1–2.6 mmol/L (8.8–10.7 mg/dL, 4.3–5.2 mEq/L) with levels greater than 2.6 mmol/L defined as hypercalcemia.

Hypercapnia: High carbon dioxide levels found in blood plasma signifying type 2 respiratory failure.

Hypertrophy (cardiac): The abnormal thickening or enlargement of the heart, causing the heart to become stiff and unable to pump effectively.

Hypoesthesia: A common side effect of various medical conditions such as MS, which manifests as a reduced sense of touch or sensation, or a partial loss of sensitivity to sensory stimuli. In everyday speech this is generally referred to as numbness.

Iatrogenic: Describes a medically induced illness or symptoms resulting from administering prescribed medication, as a side effect of drugs/treatment.

Idiopathic pulmonary fibrosis: Idiopathic pulmonary fibrosis (IPF) scars the lungs and reduces the efficiency of breathing. The build-up of scar tissue (fibrosis) causes the lungs to become stiffer and lose their elasticity and be less able to inflate and take in oxygen. IPF is a progressive condition and usually gets worse over time.

Illness trajectory: A path or line drawn to describe disease progression.

Interferon: Medication used to treat various cancers and also virus infections (e.g. chronic hepatitis B, chronic hepatitis C and MS).

Justice: Key ethical principle – to treat patients in a similar manner (equity).

Korsakoff's syndrome: A chronic memory disorder related to vitamin B-1 (thiamine) deficiency. It is generally related to alcohol misuse but can also be caused by other conditions affecting thiamine levels, such as anorexia, starvation, chronic infection and weight loss surgery.

Leadership Alliance of the Care of Dying People (LACDP): An organisation launched in the UK in 2013 following a review of the Liverpool Care Pathway (LCP) intended to provide quality palliative care based on the needs and wishes of the person and those close to them. It takes the form of five new priorities for care which have replaced the LCP.

Left bundle branch block: An abnormality in the electrical impulse through the ventricles, causing a delay in left ventricular contraction.

Macmillan holistic needs assessment: A holistic care plan that may include ideas to help patients manage emotional, physical or practical worries.

Macmillan nurses: Specialist nurses funded initially by the Macmillan charity.

Medicinal cannabis sativex (nabiximols): The first cannabis-based medicine to be licensed in the UK. The drug is prescribed for the treatment for MS-related spasticity when a person has shown inadequate response to other symptomatic treatments or found their side effects intolerable.

Mental Capacity Act 2005: Applies to everyone involved in the care, treatment and support of people aged 16 and over living in England and Wales who are unable to make all or some decisions for themselves. The MCA is designed to protect and restore power to vulnerable people who lack capacity.

Mixed dementia: A term which usually means the person has different types of dementia running concurrently. This is commonly Alzheimer's disease and vascular dementia together but can be others. Signs and symptoms of these two different types are similar but presentation and disease progression differ.

Motor neurone disease (MND): A rare progressive neurodegenerative disease that attacks the upper and lower motor neurones.

Multiple myeloma: A type of cancer which affects plasma cells.

National End of Life Care Intelligence Network: Part of Public Health England's end of life care programme aimed at improving the collection and analysis of information related to the quality, volume and costs of care provided by the NHS, social services and the third sector to adults approaching the end of life.

Neuropathic pain: Pain that develops when the nervous system is damaged due to disease or injury.

Nociceptive pain: Acute pain arising from physical damage or potential damage to the body. Examples might be the pain felt from an injury, a dental procedure or arthritis. It tends to be relieved quite quickly when treated.

Non-cognitive features of dementia: Also referred to as behavioural and psychological symptoms which relate to mood, appetite and sleep disturbance, increased anxiety, hallucinations, delusions and, for some, altered behaviours such as aggression.

Non-maleficence: Key ethical principle – do no harm (enshrined in the Hippocratic oath).

Opioid: A term for a number of natural substances (originally derived from the opium poppy) and their semisynthetic and synthetic analogues that bind to specific opioid receptors – e.g. morphine sulphate.

Opioid toxicity: The main toxic effect of opioids is decreased respiratory rate and depth, which can progress to apnoea. Other complications (e.g. pulmonary oedema) can occur, which usually develop from within minutes to a few hours after an opioid overdose. Symptoms of toxicity include pupils that are miotic, delirium, hypotension, bradycardia, decreased body temperature and urinary retention.

Pamidronate: Belongs to a group of drugs called bisphosphonates. It can be used to treat bone weakness or pain caused by myeloma and can also be used to treat high levels of calcium in the blood.

Parenteral nutrition: The provision of nutrients by an intravenous route.

Paternalism: Practice by people in authority of restricting the freedom and responsibilities of others.

Pathological grief: Also referred to as complicated grief, this is a grief reaction diagnosed 12 months after death when the bereaved person is not improving. By labelling someone's grief as pathological, a doctor is indicating that the grieving process resolution is delayed for some reason and that professional help is needed.

Percutaneous endoscopic gastronomy (PEG): PEG tubes are a minimally invasive and highly effective method for providing nutrition in patients unable to take in food by mouth for a prolonged period of time.

Peripheral neuropathy: Damage to nerves, which may impair sensation or movement, and is often in the hands and feet.

Peritoneal dialysis (PD): During PD, fluid is drained into the peritoneal cavity, allowed to sit there for several hours while it absorbs waste products and then drained out.

Personal independence payments (PIPs): Extra money to help patients with everyday life if they have an illness, disability or mental health condition.

PET scan: Positron emission tomography scans are used to produce 3D images of the inside of the body. They can be combined with CT and MRI scans. An injection of radiation is given beforehand and the scan detects this radiation in the body to produce the images.

Physician-assisted dying: Also referred to as physician-assisted suicide. The prescription or supply of drugs with the explicit intention of enabling the patient to end his or her own life (the administration of lethal drugs by both the patient and the physician is considered to be euthanasia).

Preferred place of care: Also referred to as preferred priorities of care (PPC). A hand-held patient document that helps them and their families prepare for the future end of life care.

Pregabalin: Used to treat nerve pain, epilepsy and anxiety. Nerve pain can be caused by different illnesses such as diabetes and shingles, or an injury.

Prima facia: Used to describe something which appears to be true when you first consider it.

Prognostic indicators: Assessment tools to support clinicians working with people at end of life. A prognostic indicator can help to identify/predict mortality. There are a number of tools developed for different disease areas. Commonly used for dementia are the Gold Standards Framework (GSF) and Supportive and Palliative Care Indicator Tool (SPICT).

Schwartz rounds: Schwartz rounds provide a structured forum where all staff, clinical and non-clinical, come together regularly to discuss the emotional and social aspects of working in healthcare.

Six-minute walk test: Assessment of respiratory ability. It is a sub-maximal exercise test used to assess aerobic capacity and endurance. The distance covered over a time of six minutes is used as the outcome by which to compare changes in performance capacity.

SPECT scan: Single-photon Emission Computerised Tomography is a type of nuclear imaging using radioactive substances to show how blood flows to tissues and organs.

SPIKES model: A method for disclosing sensitive information to patients using a six-step approach.

Spiritual care teams: Often members of the Church, as well as leaders from other faiths such as rabbis and imans, and humanists, who provide spiritual care within institutional settings such as hospitals and hospices.

Spirituality: Generally referred to as a subjective experience that exists both within and outside of traditional religious systems, which relates to the way in which people make sense of and understand their lives.

Stem cell transplant: A transplant of healthy stem cells which then produce normal blood cells.

Supportive care: The prevention and management of the adverse side effects of cancer and its treatment, from diagnosis through to end of life care; best supportive care indicates that no further active treatment interventions are either appropriate or offered.

Supportive/palliative care clinic: An integrated approach to enable joint reviews/ discussion to provide a coordinated, holistic approach for patients.

Surprise question: A question such as 'Would you be surprised if this patient died in the next three to six months?' used to identify patients at high risk of death who might benefit from palliative care services.

Syringe driver: Often small battery-operated devices used to administer pain relief in a patient unable to tolerate oral medication. Can include analgesia, antiemetics and other drugs. They help to reduce symptoms by delivering a steady flow of injected medication continuously under the skin. It's sometimes called a continuous subcutaneous infusion.

Terminal restlessness/delirium: Also referred to as terminal agitation, this is delirium with cognitive impairment. It tends to occur frequently at the end stages of cancer and at the end of life. The main symptoms are agitation, myoclonic jerks or twitching, irritability and impaired consciousness.

Thalidomide: Biological therapy used in combination with other drugs as part of chemotherapy treatment.

Titration (of drugs): The process of determining the medication dose that reduces symptoms to the greatest possible degree while avoiding possible side effects. When drug dosage is titrated, it is adjusted to assess how much medicine the patient requires to allow maximum effect.

Total pain management: Denotes a holistic approach to symptom management that includes physical symptoms, mental distress, social problems and emotional difficulties.

Type 1 respiratory failure: Defined as hypoxaemia (low oxygen levels in plasma).

Type 2 respiratory failure: Hypoxaemia with hypercapnia (high carbon dioxide levels, seen in patients with advanced COPD).

Watchful waiting: A period of time related to the diagnosis of dementia whereby close monitoring takes place looking for and assessing changes in behaviour and cognitive functioning which affect the person's ability to carry out daily living activities.

WHO pain ladder: A three-stage process for initiating and maintaining prescribed analgesia to enable optimal pain management.

INDEX